EMOTION
HEALED & HARNESSED

THANK YOU

Samantha and Dean

Angela Rockel for hearing what I am trying to say and making it
clearer (than I ever could) for others!

The late Dr Melissa Harte for enlightening me with
an understanding of High Sensitivity in myself and others.
She also instructed me in Emotion-Focused therapy (EFT).
Her legacy, especially with regard to EFT, is huge.

Alanna at Little Nook Creative (littlenookcreative.com)
for her cover design and advice.

Finally, a special thanks to the team at PositivePsychology.com,
especially Hugo Alberts and Seph Fontane Pennock, for creating and
making available their Emotional Intelligence Masterclass©.
It was part of my inspiration for writing this book.

EMOTION
HEALED & HARNESSED

Create the Life You Desire

*Flower Essence, Meditation and
Emotion-Focused Therapies*

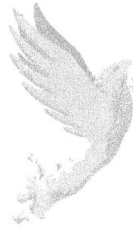

Mark Wells

Disclaimer

The information and advice contained in this book is not intended to replace the services of a qualified health professional. Consult your physician for advice. Use of the information contained herein is beyond the control of authors and publisher, who are not responsible for any problems arising from its application.

MarkVWells
P0 Box 79
Kew East, 3102
Melbourne, Australia
Telephone: 0409 985 970
Website: hsphealth.com.au

First Printing 2025 by HSP Health

Cover design (and recurring motifs) by Alanna Rance (littlenookcreative.com)

Editing and design by Angela Rockel

Printed in Australia by IngramSpark Melbourne

ISBN 978-0-646-71581-0

CONTENTS

INTRODUCTION

In my work as a naturopath, as well as from life experience and my studies, I have come to the conclusion that the key to health and wellbeing lies in the way we feel about ourselves—our overall concept of Self, the quality of our Self-consciousness. Many years ago, Rudolf Steiner became convinced that our unconscious beliefs dictate the kind of world we live in and the kind of people we become. He believed that if people really grasped this insight their world would be transformed (Gary Lachman, 2007).

The core of wellbeing lies in the relationship we have with our 'true' Self, rather than the persona-self we present to the world. That's why I give so much credence to anything that can inform us about the Self and improve our relationship with it. Flower essence therapy (FET), meditation therapy and emotion-focused therapy (EFT) all enhance emotional awareness and intelligence and also how we feel about ourselves in positive and permanent ways. Attainment of knowledge of the true Self, or Self-realisation, can be described as realisation by oneself of the opportunities offered by one's character and personality. Our unlimited potential emerges from this realisation.

Many of us still see ourselves as if through the eyes of another, from a very limited perspective, as distinct from an unlimited, holistic one that embraces all levels of being, emotional and spiritual. The lens through which we view ourselves is, sadly, also the lens through which we view our world. It is often characterised by limitations, weaknesses and an emphasis on what we lack, a lens that highlights the 'shoulds,' 'have tos' and 'must nots.' We put conditions on ourselves to be as good as we 'should' be, which is too often as good as someone else thinks we should be. We try to live up to standards and behaviours that originate from outside our Self, often from an internalised voice of a significant other such as a parent. We focus on our flaws and on all the things we are not and wish to be. The way we view ourselves is therefore conditional. If, on the other hand, we relate to ourselves unconditionally, we gain deeper self-understanding that includes recognising the signals we get from our subconscious, and so we come to perceive our own unique beauty. As Carl Jung put it, we '[discover] and satisfy our profound inherent potential.' Through our own internal sensing we feel complete and adequate as we are, and a more meaningful existence arises from this stronger sense of Self. We feel good in our own skin.

We need to view ourselves through a holistic lens that provides a multidimensional perspective on our being. If we acknowledge our weaknesses, vulnerabilities and pain, but also look deep within to shed light on our strengths and innate self-healing potentials, these adaptive qualities allow us to function at our optimum so that we can thrive: 'Who looks outside, dreams; who looks inside, awakes' (Carl Jung, *CW*).

A powerful way to broaden our view of ourselves and others is to look within and put a spotlight on our emotional nature. In this way we develop emotional intelligence—understanding our own deep emotions and those of others, using emotion-related skills and abilities such as emotional awareness for healing Self and others. Informed and enlightened by our emotions, we can express and harness them so that we perform at our optimum to create the life we desire.

These skills are essential for physical, emotional, mental and spiritual wellbeing. Viewing ourselves more deeply shifts our primary attention from what is wrong with us to what is right with us, and to the inner resources we already possess. The ability to heal and be fulfilled is innate and can be accessed, nurtured and enhanced through the practice of meditation, and the use of resources available in our natural environment such as plants, especially in their flower essence form.

My intent in this book is to hold up a holistic lens that allows you to bring into focus a multidimensional view of your Self. Through the use of practical and natural therapies such as flower essence, meditation and emotion-focused therapies, you can heal and harness your emotional

EMOTION

The knowledge of the heart is in no book
and is not to be found in the mouth of any teacher,
but grows out of you like the green seed from the dark earth.
(C.G. Jung, *The Red Book*)

For centuries, our world has placed much emphasis on the cultivation and development of our intellectual nature, but has placed less value on our emotional and spiritual nature. Education, even in the fields of psychology and sociology, has encouraged 'a fundamental imbalance caused by the excessive development of the lower, practical [thinking] mind and a simultaneous repression of the emotional [feeling] nature' (Evangelia Tsavdari, 2023). Our personal growth and development will be inhibited if we are unable to properly access what our emotional nature tells us about our basic human needs and values, and what we desire in life—our heart-felt passions.

Inner, heart-felt experience is of paramount importance—not an intellectual description of experience prescribed by another. 'Consciousness widens with [our own] attempts in language to encompass styles of thought that are adequate to [our own] experience' (Rockel, 2019). Flower essences can help us gain access to awareness.

The amount of time that children can engage in true creative play, particularly the forces of imagination and inspiration, is vastly under-cultivated in both home, community, and school environments. Modern pedagogical methods utilize intellectual methods of memory in which the brain is rapidly fired, rather than *deeper forms of memory that develop more slowly by the heart's engagement over time, including the process of forgetting and then 're-membering' and re-encountering phenomena with a freshly awakened perspective.* The modern approaches to the education of the child are particularly painful for sensitive children who are inundated with intellectual and technological forms of surface 'learning' that bypass the true longing of the heart to fully experience and engage in life-based learning. (Patricia Kaminski, 'Nurturing the heart-womb')

Integrating into a child's learning *'the heart's engagement over time, including … forgetting and then "re-membering" and re-encountering phenomena'* also teaches a child emotional resilience. A significant part of this book is devoted to natural remedies and ways to apply this approach to learning with adults who have suffered childhood and other emotional trauma. Engaging a heart-centred approach to the process of 're-membering' repressed emotional trauma can allow the wiser and more empowered adult to re-vision their experience from a freshly awakened perspective. 'Reactivation of a long-term memory returns the memory to a fragile and labile state, initiating a re-stabilisation process called *reconsolidation,* which allows for updating of the memory' (Melissa Harte, 2019). A new perspective alters the stored (original) memory, and it becomes *consolidated* as one in which survival needs—to feel safe, secure and supported—which were unmet at the time the trauma occurred, can now be met.

The development of the intellect at the expense of emotion has often been seen as a sign of evolutionary progress, despite the fact that repression of our emotional nature does not equal transcendence, deliverance or redemption (Lucis Trust, 2023). We *can* progress, though, by taking advantage of everyday opportunities, without repressing our personalities or ignoring them. Repression and avoidance will only increase the need for expression. We can achieve true progress by developing acceptance and compassion—first toward *Self,* then toward others—helped greatly along the journey through the use of flower essences, meditation and other emotion-focused therapies.

Flower essence for integrating emotions: Downy Avens (FES group)

Negative state
Precocious development of intellectual capacities
with lagging emotional development
Easily bored or distracted due to lack of
heart attention and imagination
Tendency to hyperactivity or attention deficit disorder

Positive state
Intelligence that is integrated in head and heart
Enduring wisdom derived from incremental
development of soul forces
Patient and progressive cultivation of thinking forces
with over-all soul identity (FES)

HOW EMOTIONS INFORM US

An emotion is a multi-component experience, incorporating changes in muscle tension, release of hormones, changes in cardiovascular activity, shifts in facial expression, attention, and cognition—all unfolding over a short time. An emotion is a complex state, involving many different physical and mental processes at once. From ancient times, the water element has been used as a symbol for these shifting qualities of our emotion/desire nature. Water symbolises the *layers, undercurrents and different depths* that exist in a human being, expressing the fluid ebb and flow of emotion/desire. We say that someone is swept through by desire, swept off their feet, or drowning in their sorrows. When water flows along its designated course, it is healthy and life-giving to everything in its path. But when the flow is blocked, water can become stagnant and diseased, and so can pools of unexpressed desire. We ignore, invalidate, deny or repress a felt emotion at our own peril!

If we allow our emotions to inform us, we will be able to read the meaning that exists for us in everyday experiences and events. Life is constantly communicating, imparting insight, help, and wisdom. Our emotions tell us whether important goals, values and needs are being hindered or advanced by a life situation. Emotions are a significant part of our experience of our inner and outer worlds, no matter what degree of conscious awareness we have of them. Emotions inform a person in two main ways—the first is reactive and the second is more proactive.

Emotional feedback

Firstly, emotions can give us feedback about how we are *reacting* to what's happening in and around us. This feedback can be likened to data to be assessed, informing us about ourselves now and for the future. I remember once trying to convince a very 'rational' client about the importance of emotions, and the need to acknowledge them, to feel them and to utilise them in decision making. He was convinced it was best to be as objective as possible and not let feelings have any influence over his work or personal decisions. I inadvertently struck a chord with him when I described emotions/feelings as important data to consider. As an IT data analyst by profession, he liked this analogy!

Neurobiologist Antonio Damasio (qtd. in Morse, 2006) has concluded that our emotions don't cloud our decisions but are critical to them—our emotions and decision-making ability are organically linked. He found in his patients that damage to the amygdala, which is the centre of emotions in the brain, dramatically affected their capacity for decision making. These patients were missing the emotional sentience that would make something about a decision feel good, bad, or indifferent and help them make a choice. This made it so difficult for them that they might spend hours making even the simplest decision. What we experience and how we process information is determined by the interaction between emotions (feelings that may be either in or out of our awareness), and conscious, controlled, deliberate cognition (thinking) (Harte, 2019). My client's cognitive/thinking side predominated to the point where he was suppressing, and in denial of, his emotional, feeling side. His head and heart were definitely not in harmony, and his quality of life and health were, as a consequence, being undermined. Black Eyed Susan flower essence proved very helpful for him.

Flower essence integrating heart/mind: Black Eyed Susan (FES group)

Negative state
Repressed and mentally 'edited' feelings
'Festering' emotion—'emotional boils'—a message sent
by my client's inflamed skin

Positive state
Self-awareness through 'penetrating insight' (FES)
Opening of doors to our full potential

In those who can benefit from Black Eyed Susan flower essence, it is the intellect that edits and represses what are deemed to be 'invalid' emotions. It takes huge energy to keep parts of our psyche repressed. Great resources of creativity become available when you are no longer using energy for repression, giving you a sense of vitality you may not have felt for years (Wells, *Embracing the Gift* p. 109). My client's gut and inflammatory skin conditions improved significantly after taking Black Eyed Susan flower essence, but also, he began to *feel* much better about life in general!

Interoception

The second way emotions inform us is through the subconscious and conscious mind's 'construction' of our perception of what's happening in and around us. This is a *proactive* process rather than a reactive one. Fieldman-Barrett (2017) claims: '[W]e all construct perceptions of each other's emotions' (p. 51). People perceive others as happy, sad, or angry because the brain applies each person's own emotional concepts to what they see. (In the example above, neurobiologist Antonio Damasio's clients who had suffered damage to the centre of emotions in the brain lost their ability to apply their own emotional concepts to what they saw.) 'We simulate with such speed that emotion concepts work in stealth, and it seems to us as if emotions are broadcast from the face, voice, or any other part, and we merely detect them' (p. 52).

Fieldman-Barrett elaborates on our original description of emotions being a multi-component experience by stating that emotions 'come from an ongoing process inside [us] called *interoception* … your brain's representation of all sensations from your internal organs and tissues, the hormones in your blood, and your immune system' (p. 56). The brain is often just responding to signals from our internal organs, tissues and skin. For this reason, we are not at the mercy of emotions that arise uninvited and control our behaviour. Interoceptive awareness means that we can be very much the architects of our emotional experiences.

[I]n higher animals (including humans) comes the capacity for interoception—the conscious detection and perception of sensory signals within the body and on the skin, in response to both internal (e.g., 'I'm hungry!') and external stimuli ('What's that noise?'). This is a form of perception that can be so highly developed it is sometimes referred to as the sixth sense. It is not accidental that we often use the words 'feeling' and 'emotion' interchangeably; most often, interoceptive signals are processed as sensations, but sensations are the foundation of our emotional experience of what we feel, even if we are not always fully conscious of them. (Wells, *Embracing the Gift* p. 19)

Nowadays, rather than being chased by a bear, a 'threat' might be a job interview or a social situation that makes us nervous! Our bodies don't know the difference, and so react even though we 'know' there is no threatening bear present. Many people with anxiety disorders start to panic—a process often referred to as 'catastrophising'—when they notice the interoceptive signals of stress such as rapid heartbeat, shallow, rapid breathing, tension etc. This spiral of panic is not the only response available to us, however.

Case study: Interoceptive awareness

Here is an example from my own experience. I have diverticulitis, as did my late mother. I manage it very well with natural medicines and being mindful of what I eat, but also, of what triggers it emotionally. I believe that is why I have never required medical intervention or treatment. (We will discuss the relationship of emotions to different kinds of illness in another section of the book.) Several times over the past few years, I have become aware of a phenomenon that occurs as part of my interoceptive awareness. On some occasions when I think about something I usually find stressful—an upcoming public speaking engagement or an uncomfortable social situation, for example—I feel, just for an instant, an intense sense of dread, accompanied by a painless twitching sensation in my colon. Then within 24 hours, there is always a little blood in my stool. Which comes first—the dread or the colon twitch? I am never sure. But that's where it ends—instead of panicking when I feel these interoceptive sensations, I have learned to experience them as something I can simply perceive.

According to recent understanding, we only become aware of our emotional state once we notice a change in our physical state through interoception. In the end it doesn't matter which comes first, the chicken or the egg. What we are certain of is that fear, happiness, sadness, and excitement all give physical signals within the body. Our organs are in constant communication with our brain, but usually at a subconscious level that we're not aware of. We generally won't feel our body regulating our blood pressure or blood sugar levels, but there are certain internal sensations we *are* aware of, such as fast heartbeat, shortness of breath etc. The interoceptive awareness I have in my colon probably isn't felt by most people who suffer from diverticulitis, but I'm sure this useful awareness can be developed. Being alert to my own interoceptive signals helps me to recognise my emotional state, be less likely to catastrophise, and more able to formulate a helpful response to situations as they arise. This ultimately reduces my stress levels.

In my own experience as well as with clients, highly sensitive persons (HSPs) have more highly developed interoceptive awareness than most people, and this awareness is also more intense. Interoception helps us to form our most basic sense of self. If you are unaware of, and unfamiliar with your body's signals, you're less likely to be able to regulate your emotions, and also less likely to display emotional intelligence or trust your intuition. In other words, people who are in touch with their bodies have a greater opportunity to create health and wellbeing for themselves than others who are less in touch. They have more autonomy with regard to their health (or ill-health) and wellbeing.

Mindfulness meditation is one way to develop awareness. Professor Cynthia Price at the University of Washington has been developing a new form of mindfulness that focuses on interoception. Meditation and mindfulness usually deal with becoming aware of mental experiences and quieting the mind, but Price's method also brings focus to interoceptive sensations in the body. Having noted this, most 'scripts' for progressive muscle relaxation (PMR) and mindfulness involve, at some point early in the process, a focused awareness on what's happening inside one's body, and of interoceptive sensations in the moment.

A good example of interoceptive awareness occurs for most of us when we are driving a car. Often when we have had a 'near miss' such as a narrowly avoided collision or other accident, we drive on and then notice that our heart is beating faster, our stomach muscles remain braced and there is tension in other areas of the body. If we don't manage to calm down and ease these sensations, the next far less threatening experience is likely to feel as panic-inducing as the previous near miss. We are more likely to catastrophise because interoceptive signals from the near miss are still being sent to our brain, telling us that not only are we still under threat, but now another threat has been added! In this situation, Nectarine flower essence can help.

Flower essence for calm after a crisis: Nectarine (FES group)

Negative state
For 'riders of the storm'
Anxious feelings of life being out of one's control

Positive state
The 'calm after the storm'
Restored faith and TRUST

Nectarine flower essence helps us recover composure and calm, heart-centred consciousness in the midst of or just after a crisis, restoring our faith and trust, and helping us to become more peaceful and emotionally balanced (Wells, *Essential Flower Essence Book* p. 255).

Effects of FE therapy and meditation on mood and emotion

Although the words emotion and mood are often used interchangeably, they are closely related but distinct phenomena with the following differences. Firstly, emotions are typically short-lived, while moods are more long-lasting. Whereas emotions usually come on instantly and subside quickly, moods often develop slowly and take time to change. You could say that if an emotion lasts, it has developed into a mood. (I often watched this transformation occur right before my eyes in my children during their teens!) Secondly, people can usually specify the event associated with experiencing an emotion—it has a clear trigger such as an argument with a friend, receiving a compliment, or successful completion of a task.

In contrast, a mood is more free-floating and can occur without apparent cause (Brehm, 1999). I have always had what I call 'dark' days and nights that seemingly come out of the blue (excuse the pun!), and perhaps at these times the subconscious is downloading from my 'shadow' side, as Carl Jung called it. Moods may also occur as a result of an accumulation of events and experiences. And finally, emotions are hard to miss—they are front of mind while moods typically sit at the back of the mind, and from there have a big influence on emotions. If someone gets into their car in a 'bad mood' they will be more likely to experience a flash of angry emotion if another car cuts in on them.

Flower essences have a direct positive influence on our moods, as will be described in case studies throughout this book. Here is a summary of some research I carried out, which investigated the influence of a

Bach Flower essence combination called Rescue Remedy™ (RR) on mood in forty-four women aged between 18 and 40 who were taking no other mood treatment medication. In a double-blind, cross-over, placebo-based trial, the Profile of Mood States (POMS) test was used to assess the moods of all participants. POMS is a standard psychological questionnaire that asks you to choose from a list of 65 words/statements to indicate how you have been feeling.

The 'cross-over' aspect of the trial involved giving the same person both placebo and Rescue Remedy at different times and comparing the effects. This is the procedure that is followed in situations where each person's response is very subjective. For example, it is used in pain management trials—there is no point in comparing how a substance affects the pain of two different people, because everyone has a different pain threshold, so it is necessary to give each individual both the substance and a placebo.

My Bach Flower essence trial compared how a person responded to a placebo compared with how the same person responded to Rescue Remedy. The trial was conducted over seven weeks. Each participant received either Rescue Remedy or a placebo for the first three weeks, followed by a one week 'wash-out' period without taking either mixture. After the wash-out period, they were 'crossed over' and allocated the placebo mixture if they had previously received Rescue Remedy and vice versa. As in all double-blind trials, neither I nor the participants had any knowledge of whether they were being given placebo or Rescue Remedy. *Significant POMS overall score differences resulted between placebo and RR treatment, and the greatest difference was found when 'tension/anxiety' scores were isolated* (Wells, *Essential Flower Essence Book* p. 24).

Like flower essences, meditation can also have a positive effect on mood and emotion. While meditating, the mind relaxes and calms so deeply that emotions and moods lose their influence. We surrender to a *calm, natural ease and stillness within*—in other words we connect with the true Self that is unaffected by emotions and moods. The more we practise meditation the more easily we can access this inner sense of natural quiet and ease.

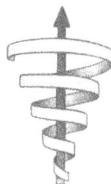

PRIMARY EMOTIONS: ADAPTIVE AND MALADAPTIVE RESPONSES

Primary emotions are peoples' first, gut-feeling responses to what is going on inside and outside of them. We are all born equipped with an adaptive emotion system, responsible for instinctive responses that we rely on to survive and thrive. Primary emotions are direct, unmediated reactions to events, and they can be used to communicate our intentions to others (Izard, 1990). Primary emotions need to be attended to, validated and acted upon at the time they arise. There are seven primary emotions identified as universal across cultures (Izard, 1977):

- happiness/joy
- anger
- sadness
- fear
- disgust
- interest, surprise or curiosity
- shame

Primary emotions are often characterised as either positive (happiness, joy, interest, curiosity) or negative (fear, sadness, anger, shame), but this can be misleading because, depending on the situation, any emotion can impact in a positive or negative way. They are pure and unadulterated by prior emotions or cognitions and can be either adaptive or maladaptive. Greenberg (2024, p. 6) states: '[T]hey orient us to the environment and provide good information. Adaptive emotions fit the activating situation and help a person to cope with it.' They organise the individual for adaptive action and help them get their needs met (Frijda, 1986). In Traditional Chinese Medicine no emotion is viewed as 'bad' or negative; it only becomes a problem when we become stuck in an emotion or skip over or avoid an emotion.

Anger, for instance, is an essential emotion that can be empowering in some situations, for example when it helps us to access the assertiveness needed to 'draw the line' and declare that a personal boundary has been crossed, or that we are being hurt or harmed. Not only does it inform us when limits have been crossed but also reminds us of where our values lie, and when expressed wisely and creatively, can be a powerful force for change. In this way anger can be *adaptive*. However, in some circumstances anger can take over a person's life. Whether acted upon or suppressed, it can cause tremendous suffering, can lead to loss of jobs and relationships, and can leave individuals feeling ashamed, powerless, and alone. In this way anger can be *maladaptive*.

Fear is positive/adaptive when it narrows our focus to a specific threat in our environment and keeps us safe. It helps us to take direct action to escape the threat and remain vigilant when necessary. But if intense fear persists it can become negative/maladaptive in its impact if this narrowing of focus paralyses us. When this happens, we lose perspective, and this hampers our ability to act in the interest of our own wellbeing and quality of life. A constant, underlying feeling of panic/fear also increases levels of cortisol (stress hormone), suppressing our immune system and making us more vulnerable and less able to adapt to infection and ill-health. This is an important point to recognise when the world is in panic/fear mode—as we saw in response to a pandemic!

Curiosity can be positive/adaptive in that it can help us discover exciting and useful things, and can help us to observe and perceive difficult emotions/thoughts differently, so that they have less negative impact on us. However, we also know that 'curiosity killed the cat'! Rather than saying emotions are 'good' or 'bad,' or positive or negative, for most situations a better way of categorising them would be to describe them as *adaptive* or *maladaptive* depending on a person's situation and experience. This way, an emotion can be adaptive in one situation and maladaptive in another. So-called negative emotions can be adaptive and so-called positive emotions can be maladaptive.

Adaptive functions of emotions

- Happiness/joy—broadens the scope of attention to provide more options, including desired and creative actions; increases a person's sense of unity and ability to work cooperatively
- Anger—mobilises action to defend one's boundaries (when violated), leading to assertiveness and empowerment
- Sadness—mobilises action to seek comfort, or withdrawal to process grief; enables healing and adaptation to loss
- Fear—plays a vital role in survival when it narrows attention to mobilise the fight or flight response to a current threat
- Disgust—mobilises action to evacuate or withdraw from a toxic person or experience
- Interest, surprise or curiosity—expands a person's openness to new experiences, broadens one's mind
- Shame—mobilises action to hide or temporarily retreat from the scrutiny of others, to reassess then adaptively respond

Maladaptive emotions

A primary emotion is 'the emotion that a person might feel first when confronted with a particular situation or might be suppressed if it was unsafe to express it' (Harte, 2019, p. 21). If a primary emotion is not acted upon, for example as a result of trauma or neglect when we do not manage to engage and respond, our emotional system malfunctions and complex, maladaptive emotions and responses evolve as a result. '[M]aladaptive emotions differ from primary adaptive emotions in that they are chronic dysfunctional feelings that originally [may have been] adaptive responses to bad situations but are currently no longer adaptive' (Greenberg, 2024, p. 6). They may have served their purpose at the time to protect a person from further physical abuse, for instance. However, now they are reactions to the past in the present, and do not help people cope adaptively to the current situation or allow the original unmet needs to be satisfied.

In emotion-focused therapy (EFT), the original unacted primary emotion or trauma response, which may have been suppressed or invalidated, is re-attended to, validated and acted upon with the support of a therapist. Other emotional-focused therapies such as flower essence therapy and meditation also allow a person to work through and better act upon their primary emotions rather than suppress or ignore them. According to Elliot et al. (2004) there are three types of emotions that are maladaptive, with associated dysfunctional behaviour.

1. Primary maladaptive emotional responses: If primary emotions are not expressed and acted upon adaptively in response to traumatic experiences at the time they occur, '[p]eople become stuck in these emotions for months or even years' (Harte, 2019 p. 25). Maladaptive emotions are direct reactions to past (and even long past) situations—they no longer help the person cope constructively in the present. One example may be someone who regularly feels intense anxiety, fear or panic in response to something seemingly harmless in their environment. Their inability to self-regulate consistently fails and they feel confused and overwhelmed without being conscious of why. Another example: children who were often humiliated by a parent and made to feel ashamed of expressing primary feeling responses (see Pink Monkeyflower flower essence below) often experience maladaptive responses of shame or humiliation as adults, reverting to their 'default' mode, withdrawing and hiding, and/ or always deferring to others or being overly needy.

Flower essence for emotional courage: Pink Monkeyflower (FES group)

Pink Monkeyflower flower essence can help a person overcome a self-denigrating sense of shame and unworthiness about the feelings they wish to express. The flower essence allows a person to display 'emotional transparency [and the] courage to take emotional risks with others' (FES).

Negative state
Feelings of shame, guilt, or unworthiness
Fear of exposure and rejection due to prior abuse or trauma

Positive state
Emotional transparency
Courage to take emotional risks with others (FES)
(Wells, *Essential Flower Essence Book* p. 398)

2. Secondary reactive emotions: These are overtly expressed emotions that are 'reactions to, or defences against, a primary emotion or thought' (Harte, 2019 p. 25). They often 'protect us against primary emotions that are experienced as intolerable' (Greenberg, 2024 p. 7), as for example, when a child living in an extremely traumatic life situation—a war zone for instance—is so traumatised by the experience that they disassociate. They disconnect or detach from reality because their emotional pain is intolerable. It is a coping or defence mechanism to minimise pain and stress. In the immediate sense it is adaptive but going forward in the child's life it becomes extremely maladaptive, as unresolved emotional pain can be at the root of much dysfunctional behaviour.

Secondary reactive emotions hide what a person is really feeling, and therefore don't bring relief, or if they do it is short-lived, unlike the expression of primary, underlying emotions. For example, some people cry when they are actually angry. A skilled therapist who knows a client well will recognise this situation and encourage them to express the underlying anger when processing trauma. I remember attending a personal growth course in the early nineteen-eighties where participants had the opportunity to experience a cathartic release of primary emotion in relation to parental issues. Experienced facilitators encouraged participants not to collapse into an expression of secondary emotion through a submissive posture and weeping, but rather to remain upright in a more empowered stance and express their underlying anger. Pillows were close by for participants to unleash their anger on, and often took a pounding. Some ripped up an old phone book!

In this situation there was an understanding that there were layers of emotion and that it was important for healing and personal growth to get in touch with the deepest, primary layers, and to acknowledge and express them. Though the approach taken in that long-ago workshop is seldom used in therapy these days, I must admit that over the years, I have often found a few minutes with the punching bag at the gym quite cathartically therapeutic in getting rid of built-up tension, anger and frustration! Another example of secondary reactive emotion is defensiveness and hostility as a cover for underlying primary fear or sadness. Most of us know people who find it difficult to show vulnerability or even grief but instead find it easier to become aggressively defensive. In this situation Fuchsia flower essence can be useful.

Flower essence for expression of emotion: Fuchsia (FES group)

Fuchsia flower essence can help a person who is often over-reactive and displays hyper-emotionality that masks more deep-seated emotion or pain. These *superficial*, but habitual, maladaptive and dysfunctional emotions and behaviours are associated with *underlying* (unacted upon) primary emotion.

Negative state
Psychosomatic symptoms resulting from emotional repression (FES)
'False states of emotionality' (FES); 'over the top' reactions

Positive state
Deep awareness/Self-understanding
Genuine (primary) emotional expression; grounded
(Wells, *Essential Flower Essence Book* p. 184)

Meditation for emotional awareness

Along with flower essence therapy, other emotion-focused therapies such as meditation are a wonderful adjunct. Used together, they offer much more than the sum of their parts! A mindful approach to life can be developed by regularly practising meditation. This deepens our general awareness, including emotional awareness. By living more in the NOW, we can have more self-understanding of our basic, instinctual, and primary emotional responses. There is a clearer option to express the genuine Self and its needs.

3. Instrumental or manipulative emotional responses: In the third kind of maladaptive response, 'people strategically enact an emotion to get their needs met, or influence others, and usually, this process is automatic, without awareness. ... [T]he display of emotions [is] independent of the person's original [primary] emotional response to the situation' (Harte, 2019 p. 25). Let's take an example from the animal kingdom. When a dog is scared or intimidated by a bigger or more aggressive dog, it may roll over to display subservience in response to its primary emotional response of fear. It does this to pacify the more aggressive dog. It is an instinctive and automatic response that is enacted to protect itself from harm—and thus it is adaptive.

In human beings there are many common examples of instrumental emotions—a person may display anger and aggression in order to intimidate someone into doing what they want them to do. Bullying in the school playground often stems from an underlying fear in the bully. Instrumental emotions 'are essentially an indirect way of getting what one wants, without having to experience the vulnerability of making direct requests or showing primary feelings. They often backfire in the long run, and do not result in good relationships' (Greenberg, 2024 p. 8). Relationships are stressed because the people subjected to these instrumental behaviours often feel manipulated, or worse, they feel fearful and powerless when anger and aggression is directed at them.

Another common manipulative approach is where someone expresses sadness or helplessness to evoke a caring response from another without having to ask for it. In this situation, Fairy Lantern flower essence can be very helpful. Kaminski and Katz (FES) describe how 'the soul who needs Fairy Lantern still clings to a childlike personality. ... Such a person learns that she or he will receive love only by remaining in an arrested, over-dependent, childlike state.'

Case study: Arrested development

In my *Essential Flower Essence Book* I describe a client who displayed these childlike characteristics. 'Jenny' came to her first consultation accompanied by her mother, and her main concern—or I should say her mother's main concern—was a delayed and irregular menstrual cycle. Although she was nineteen, Jenny had only experienced two periods, the first when she was fifteen and the second a year and a half later after beginning hormone treatment prescribed by her doctor.

Talking to Jenny, I felt that I was talking to someone in her early teens or younger. She dressed and spoke like her mother, to whom she constantly deferred. Their relationship appeared more like that of an older sibling with a baby sister than mother and daughter. To her credit, Jenny's mother had come to realise that this co-dependent relationship was dysfunctional and was now consciously working to change it.

Jenny was struggling with two directly related issues—stifled personal growth and delayed hormonal development. Her emotional immaturity and presentation as someone much younger may have helped her *instrumentally* in the past to get some needs met but it was not serving her in the same way anymore. She was now less able to conceal her real feelings and manipulate her mother's responses. Jenny took Fairy Lantern flower essence over the next few months, and this supported the considerable personal development I observed over that time, including the natural establishment of a regular menstrual cycle. Ingrained habits take time to change, and it was an uncomfortable process to move out of what had become her comfort zone. Despite this, many of her childlike displays of emotion and behaviour disappeared and a more confident and independent young woman emerged. She reached a new level of maturity and healthy independence from her mother, who was very supportive of these changes, despite the fact that she was also being challenged to let go of a long-established co-dependency.

Flower essence for developmental maturity: Fairy Lantern (FES group)

Negative state
Delayed or 'splintered' body/mind/spirit development
'Immaturity … childish dependency' (FES)

Positive state
Balanced body/mind/spirit development
Maturity, independence, creative expression
(Wells, *Essential Flower Essence Book* p. 179)

Coexistence of opposite emotions—dual occupancy

Another thing to consider is that distinctly opposing positive and negative emotions can coexist. Negative events in our lives are associated with increases in what are generally regarded as negative emotions (e.g. fear), but they are not necessarily accompanied by decreases in positive emotions (e.g. joy). Likewise, positive events are strongly linked with increases in positive emotions, but not necessarily with decreases in negative emotions (Gable et al., 2000). A familiar example is when a young child might experience fear and overwhelm as well as joy at their birthday party, celebrated with lots of family and friends.

Research on the effects of the World Trade Centre attacks showed that the experience of positive emotions does not automatically imply the absence of negative emotions or vice versa (Fredrickson et al., 2003). More resilient personalities were found to experience fewer depressive symptoms, and they experienced positive emotions more frequently after the attacks. One man, for example, miraculously escaped the building but his friends and colleagues were killed. He felt traumatised, and sad about the loss of close friends, and even some guilt around the fact that he was spared. However, he also felt joy, and was happy to be alive, and extremely grateful. In his capacity to experience negative and positive emotions at the same time, he displayed resilience and recovered well.

There are many other examples of the existence of this duality where two qualities/aspects, often opposites, coexist within the mind and body. For example, at the level of the mind we have Carl Jung's anima and animus, feminine and masculine, introversion and extroversion, right-brain attributes and left-brain attributes, and Yin and Yang from Traditional Chinese Medicine. An example on a physical level would be the acid-alkaline balance in one's system. The phenomenon of positive and negative emotions coexisting is analogous to what happens in nature, where we can see what seem to be adaptive and maladaptive qualities coexisting in plants, as the following section will show.

Prescribing flower essences using plant signatures

The *signature* of a plant—*what its outer form and function tells us about its inner nature*—has been essential in informing traditional plant use, and has also often provided part of the reasoning behind scientific research into potential therapeutic plant use. When viewing the *signature* of a plant we observe qualities that could be regarded as weaknesses or vulnerabilities—maladaptations—but which actually work adaptively for the plant. In FET, specific signs and characteristics of a plant's form and function, especially in relation to its flower, can inform us of its healing potential for humans.

In my flower essence books and those of many other FET practitioners, each flower essence is described in terms of the negative or maladaptive human vulnerabilities and weaknesses it can help to address, and the positive or adaptive human qualities it represents and fosters. When a person takes a well-chosen flower essence, maladaptive behaviours and responses can be transformed into the innate positive potential that is expressed by the plant.

The *prime indication of suitability* when choosing a flower essence is that the plant signature has features that could symbolise the weaknesses and vulnerabilities of the person for whom the flower essence is being chosen, but which work for the plant in an adaptive way. Flower essences can help a person to cultivate the innate potential of characteristics that have previously been expressed in maladaptive ways, so that they become a source of strength and resilience. St John's Wort and Pink Yarrow flower essences are classic examples.

Flower essence for receptivity: St John's Wort (FES group)

Negative/maladaptive state
Feeling vulnerable and exposed; 'deep fears' (FES)
Disturbed sleep/dreams (FES)

Positive/adaptive state
Confident, secure, *open*-minded
Radiant and light-hearted; receptive

St John's Wort loves dry and sunny positions, and the upright stem branches at the top so that each flower can get the sun. The flower petals tend to curl back, so as to gain *maximum exposure* to the sun. 'If you look at the leaf in the sunlight it looks like it's filled with thousands of little pin-pricks. These are actually oil glands, and they leave translucent holes in the chlorophyll of the leaf, absorbing light, sort of "pulling it in"' (FES). This *perforated aspect* of the plant's signature also points to the flower essence's ability to heal holes in the human etheric body. The nervous system is the main physical link with the etheric body, so it is not surprising that the homeopathic medicine made from St John's Wort—Hypericum—is used for treating nerves that have been damaged as a result of trauma or medical procedures (Wells, *Essential Flower Essence Book* p. 302).

Those who can benefit from St John's Wort flower essence may feel sensitive, uneasy and vulnerable within themselves, as if they are too open and exposed, with an inexplicable sense of dread. This can affect their sleep, and they may experience disturbances and night terrors. A major aspect of the plant's signature relates to the way in which a person's maladaptive experience of vulnerability and feeling '*too open and exposed*' corresponds to an *adaptive* quality in St John's Wort—its *unique receptivity to the sun's healing rays*. St John's Wort can help us transform our *sense of vulnerability* into a comfortable *receptiveness* to the positive and dynamic elements in our environment. (The herbal form of St John's Wort can cause slight over-sensitivity to the sun's rays, but NOT the flower essence form.)

Flower essence for appropriate boundaries: Pink Yarrow (FES group)

Negative state
Overly sympathetic—'psychic sponge'
Lacking emotional boundaries (FES)

Positive state
'Self-contained consciousness' (FES) while maintaining empathy
Emotional clarity (Wells, *Essential Flower Essence Book* p. 276)

Pink Yarrow is another example of a flower essence that can allow vulnerability to transform into innate, adaptive strength. Several species of yarrow are used as flower essences and their signatures all relate to yarrow's herbal use since ancient times to stop wounds bleeding. These essences stop us from bleeding on an energetic level by helping to seal, protect and stabilise the life force. Yarrow flowers are arranged in finely detailed geometric patterns, interwoven to form strong, enduring structures. The colour of Pink Yarrow signifies its relationship with the heart chakra and its protective qualities as an emotional buffer so that emotional boundaries become better defined (Wells, *Essential Flower Essence Book* pp. 277, 372–73).

Because of these qualities, many therapists take Pink Yarrow flower essence—myself included! Therapists are often very open and empathetic, but this may be due to their overly permeable emotional and energetic boundaries. Their sensitivity and receptivity to clients gives them the ability to understand and empathise, and in this respect it functions as an adaptive strength. However, sensitivity can also make us very vulnerable. I have always felt that my high sensitivity is a gift and a distinct advantage in my work as a therapist—but it is also my 'Achilles heel'! We therapists cannot fully utilise the strength of our sensitivity if we are continually losing energy to others and absorbing the negative emotions of those around us. When this happens we can easily become overwhelmed and suffer burnout when our natural energetic immunity fails. Many therapists identify with the myth of Chiron, the wounded healer, who displays this fusion of maladaptive wounding and adaptive healing qualities. For me and many other therapists, Pink Yarrow flower essence helps to protect against potential vulnerability while allowing our strengths of sensitivity and depth of perception to remain intact.

Developing inner resources: The phoenix effect

Regular practice of meditation enables you to reach a level of *acceptance* of feelings/emotions, however 'bad,' threatening or negative they appear. While the mind is in a state of *natural ease and stillness*—engaging with the true Self—it becomes easier to sit with emotions and experience them without causing harm to yourself or others. All types of emotion—positive/adaptive and negative/maladaptive—can comfortably coexist when we perceive them as just part of our experience within a much wider and more resilient Self. Maladaptive emotions lose their negative impact when we relate to them in this way. In mindfulness meditation, by being present with a feeling or emotion and observing it with objective curiosity, a person detaches from it but is still able to be informed by it.

As part of my placement experience while completing my Master of Social Science degree in Counselling at Swinburne University, I worked at the outpatient department of a large hospital. While there I co-facilitated mindfulness meditation group sessions for chronic pain management. Everyone is aware of the many negative feelings associated with chronic pain—the panic when pain starts to intensify, the sense of anger and frustration, the feelings of powerlessness and hopelessness. However, regular practice of mindfulness meditation reduces our emotional reactivity to pain, and this in turn reduces the suffering associated with it (Perlman et al., 2010).

For many chronic pain sufferers, the first hint of pain after a period of being pain free often leads to what is referred to as 'catastrophising'—expecting that the pain will inevitably become intense again, which increases the likelihood that this will happen. Part of catastrophising is a 'tensing of our body in response to a primary pain and also an associated anxiety or anger or other negative mental state of non-acceptance' (McKenzie and Hassed, 2012 p. 131). Patients who become practised in mindfulness meditation develop a greater *acceptance* of their pain and so are less reactive to the first signs of its return. This circumvents catastrophising. And each time the pain passes without escalating, they become more confident that 'no sensation—not even pain … is permanent' (McKenzie and Hassed, 2012 p. 139). They come to *accept* different degrees of pain without catastrophising.

Most patients who keep up their mindfulness practice experience a significant drop in the amount of pain medication they require, and in a few cases, patients are eventually able to stop pain medication completely. In such cases, the individual has reached a level of acceptance that enables them to remain conscious of discomfort or background pain while moving through their normal day with a greater sense of inner calm and ease. I recall one client putting it this way: 'Before, if my pain flared up, I would freak out and get really stressed, which only made the pain worse. Now I'm able to keep myself calm as long as I keep doing my mindfulness meditation.' The amount of pain medication she required dropped dramatically. She acknowledged that it was 'still a work in progress' but believed she had taken a big step towards reclaiming her life from the grip of constant pain.

The positive feelings/emotions induced by meditation practice are adaptive, enabling people to maintain a broader perspective so that positive feelings outweigh negative feelings. They become aware of being *much more* than their pain, which recedes somewhat into the background. Throughout this book I give examples of how, despite emotionally traumatic experiences as a child, adolescent or adult, people can recover and show great resilience, like a phoenix rising from the ashes. They can heal and become the person they desire to be!

The *broadening effect* of positive/adaptive emotions (Frederickson & Branigan, 2005) significantly lessens and '*undoes*' the impact of negative/maladaptive emotions associated with pain (Frederickson et al., 2000), which, though they continue, are relegated to the background. Love-Lies-Bleeding flower essence is helpful for maintaining this adaptive response to chronic pain.

Flower essence for adaptive emotion: Love-Lies-Bleeding (FES group)

Negative state

Intensification of pain and suffering due to isolation

Profound melancholia or despair due to over-personalising one's pain

Positive state

Transcendent consciousness

Ability to move beyond personal pain, suffering or mental anguish

Transpersonal vision; compassionate acceptance of life karma. (FES)

In an essay on this essence, Patricia Kaminsky says: 'Learning to accept, endure, and be with pain and suffering is often—counter-intuitively—the very process that can actually lessen such agony' (FES). Love-Lies-Bleeding flower essence helps us come to terms with our lot in life, not in a resigned way but with a compassionate and transpersonal understanding of our suffering and discomfort. Rather than feeling isolated and alone in our struggle with pain, it enables us to sense how our burden is lightened when shared with our direct karmic connections and the rest of the world (FES). We are able to put physical and mental anguish in a broader perspective, understanding that there is more to us than our pain. We no longer identify with it completely, and can recognise our own and others' pain with compassion rather than be a slave to it (Wells, *Essential Flower Essence Book* p. 392).

'NEGATIVE' EMOTIONS AND THE DISEASE MODEL OF HEALTH

Society encourages us to avoid 'negative' emotions by whatever means possible, whether by taking a pill, indulging in escapism or just turning away from anything that may cause even slight discomfort. This remains the case despite knowing that these emotions can also be adaptive and have much to teach us. Many of us still think that by fighting or fixing, ignoring, avoiding or denying feelings and emotions we have labelled negative, we can simply make them go away, and so live happily ever after. Psychological research has also focused on negative emotions and what is wrong with us, and given too little attention to our inner potential and what is right about us. Relatively little research has been focused on the factors that lift our spirits, enhance resilience and promote wellbeing. This focus on what's wrong with us—the signs/symptoms of mental or physical illness—has been referred to as the *disease model* of health and human functioning. The disease model is explained in Fig. 1 below.

Figure I: Primary focus on repairing weakness—the disease model of health

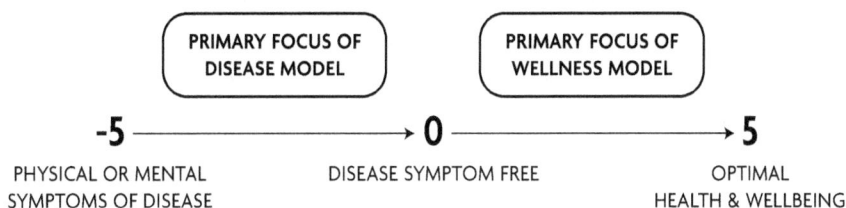

```
┌──────────────────────┐        ┌──────────────────────┐
│   PRIMARY FOCUS OF   │        │   PRIMARY FOCUS OF   │
│    DISEASE MODEL     │        │    WELLNESS MODEL    │
└──────────────────────┘        └──────────────────────┘

   -5 ──────────────────────→ 0 ──────────────────────→ 5
PHYSICAL OR MENTAL         DISEASE SYMPTOM FREE           OPTIMAL
SYMPTOMS OF DISEASE                               HEALTH & WELLBEING
```

In this picture, –5 represents suffering from mental or physical health problems, 0 represents not suffering from these problems, and +5 represents wellbeing and thriving. The disease model is focused on the –5 to 0 section. Therapeutic interventions are designed to move people from –5 to 0, reducing distressing symptoms and dysfunctionality, and hopefully preventing relapse. The end goal (0-point) is achieved when a person is no longer experiencing diagnosable symptoms of mental or physical illness.

In the broader context of health, work and performance, a weakness focus means that our prime concern is symptoms and behaviours that are causing suboptimal health or low performance. In a clinical context for a health practitioner, this means that the focus is predominantly on signs and symptoms of illness. Once these symptoms are diagnosed, treated and alleviated and 0-point (Fig. 1) is reached, it is assumed that we automatically achieve overall health and wellbeing at +5. However, this does NOT necessarily follow. Also, when we focus primarily on people's weaknesses, we may ignore their existing natural, innate recuperative powers, their constitutional strengths, and the resources they possess already that promote wellbeing and resilience. These are the qualities that help us to get to +5 while preventing us from relapsing to the 0 point or below. The weakness focus only takes in part of the whole view of a person.

Once upon a time, I was supervising naturopathic students in their final year at a natural therapies college in Melbourne. One student, who also happened to be a qualified medical doctor, said to me: 'I find I have to do two separate consultations, one after the other, every time I see a client here at the student clinic. The first is my 15-minute medical consultation in which I concentrate on physical illness symptoms and eliminate anything that needs urgent medical attention. The second consultation starts immediately after, when I put on my naturopath hat and take a more holistic view of the client in front of me.' He found that not only was the standard 15-minute medical consultation too short a time to develop a holistic physical, emotional and mental view of the person, but that even without a time constraint (at least an hour was allowed for the naturopathic consults), he had to compartmentalise the two views of the patient and put on a different 'hat' for each. This experience highlights some of the deficits of the disease model.

Five misconceptions fostered by the disease model

The disease model has been used for a long time as the dominant approach to physical health by many researchers and practitioners, but more preventative and holistic treatments and approaches are emerging. In mental health research also, an awareness of some important misconceptions associated with the disease model has led to a more holistic view. This is especially true in the area of Positive Psychology, which includes a better understanding of good health and wellbeing (0 to +5 on the Fig. 1 scale), and how we achieve and maintain it. Material presented here is based on the Positive Psychology Program at PositivePsychology.com.

Misconception #1: If you fix what is wrong, you will automatically achieve health and wellbeing

Underlying the weakness focus of the disease model is the belief that fixing what is wrong will automatically establish wellbeing. However, getting rid of anger, fear, and depression will not automatically lead to peace, love, and joy. Getting to the 0 point on the scale in Fig. 1 doesn't automatically lead you to +5 on the scale. Strategies to reduce fear, anger, or depression are not identical to strategies that maximise peace, joy, or a sense of meaning. Wellbeing is not merely the absence of negative emotion, but more importantly, it is the presence of positive emotion.

'Negative' emotion, flower essence therapy and meditation

In flower essence therapy, negative emotions are acknowledged but not solely targeted to be eliminated. A flower essence is prescribed to enable a person to move from a state that foregrounds their maladaptive emotions towards a better balance with more adaptive emotions. In meditation, one can reach a level of acceptance of 'negative' thoughts and feelings. They are not eliminated but have decidedly less impact. As the mind becomes more naturally at-ease and calm, more positive thoughts and feelings begin to prevail. Research shows that the absence of mental illness does not imply the presence of mental wellbeing, nor does the presence of mental illness imply the absence of mental wellbeing (Westerhope & Keyes, 2010; Keyes et al., 2008; Lamers et al., 2011). There are people who suffer from psychological or physical disorders, who still experience subjective wellbeing, and conversely, there are people who report low levels of subjective wellbeing who don't suffer from any psychological or physical disorders.

Misconception #2: If you reduce your negative states, you will cope well with life

So many of us believe that if we just get rid of everything that makes us feel bad, we will cope well and live happily ever after! This isn't necessarily the case. Typically, psychological interventions aim to reduce aversive states such as negative emotions or stress. Consistent with the disease model, this aim is based on the assumption that if we reduce our aversive states, effective coping, fewer problems and enhanced wellbeing will automatically follow. For instance, stress eating or emotional eating is a maladaptive behavioural response to stress for many people with weight problems. But studies (see below) have shown that people can effectively cope and avoid weight problems, even without reduction of stress, negative emotions or other aversive states. It is therefore not the absence of stress that brings about successful weight maintenance, but rather the ability to effectively deal with stress. This has implications for all weight-loss dieting. If, along with dietary advice, the person doesn't receive counselling and guidance about ways to improve their ability to effectively manage stress, they are likely to fail.

Kristeller and Wolever (2011) found that mindfulness meditation helped people manage their varying emotional responses, and improved their ability to emotionally self-regulate in the presence of stress factors. As a consequence, they were able to make better food choices and develop better awareness of their hunger and when they had eaten enough. It is not necessarily the experience of stress that negatively impacts on our health, but the way we deal with perceived stress. The way people deal with and perceive difficult experiences, rather than their occurrence, is the best indication of successful coping.

An interesting connection can be drawn here with the assertion, first made in the 19th century by practitioners of the 'Nature Cure' (now referred to as naturopathy): 'It is not the germ, it is the soil.' If you get the soil right, it will cope with pathogens it is exposed to. A modern interpretation of this principle is that the state of our overall health and wellbeing decides how successfully or otherwise we deal with bacteria and viruses. If we are in good enough health, our susceptibility is normal and our natural immunity will act to effectively protect against and/or manage pathogens that have the potential to cause harm or disease. From this perspective where we shift the focus to ourselves and our ability to manage stress, the perception of outside influences changes, including how we view external stressors.

Research into post-traumatic recovery—the development and maintenance of a positive outlook following trauma—further supports the idea that it is not merely a reduction in negative states but the presence of positive states that reflects effective coping. Positive changes may include a different way of relating to others, awareness of personal strengths ('what doesn't kill you makes you stronger'), spiritual changes, and increased appreciation of life (Tedeschi and Calhoun, 2009). Any therapy that can support and help us take the view that difficulties, challenges and stresses are also opportunities for personal growth will significantly increase our ability to cope. Scotch Broom flower essence supports this outlook.

Flower essence for adaptive responsiveness: Scotch Broom (FES group)

Negative state
Discouraged and disheartened
Pessimism about the world (FES)

Positive state
Seeing difficulties/challenges as opportunities for growth
'Positive and optimistic feelings about the world' (FES)
(Wells, *Essential Flower Essence Book* pp. 308–09)

In the negative or maladaptive state of mind, those who can benefit from Scotch Broom flower essence 'seem to focus on the darker side of the world psyche. The obstacles in our lives seem too big to overcome and we wonder whether there is any point to the struggle, when another obstacle is sure to be just around the corner. ... What's the use? Why try? ... Scotch Broom flower essence helps us see the challenges of life as opportunities for growth and development' (FES).

Meditation and negative emotion
The practice of meditation helps us change our perspective on negative thoughts and feelings associated with our stresses. We get better at

separating them from our true, broader-minded Self so that we can view them with more objectivity and understanding. We accept their presence because they no longer have the negative impact they once had. We manage, cope and deal better with life irrespective of whether we are subjected to stress or other aversive states.

Another example of how post-traumatic growth can serve as an effective way of coping with adversity, even without reduction of emotional pain, is found in a person who has experienced loss. The *expectation* may be that, after grieving for a time, the pain of one's loss (as represented by the dark area in Fig. 2) may fade into insignificance. However, the *reality* is more that the pain remains in existence, but one grows 'bigger and stronger' than the pain to the point where it has far less negative impact. Personal growth after an experience of adversity such as a tragic loss is not the absence of post-traumatic pain from grief, and this realisation helps us to move forward in life.

Figure 2: Grief expectation and reality

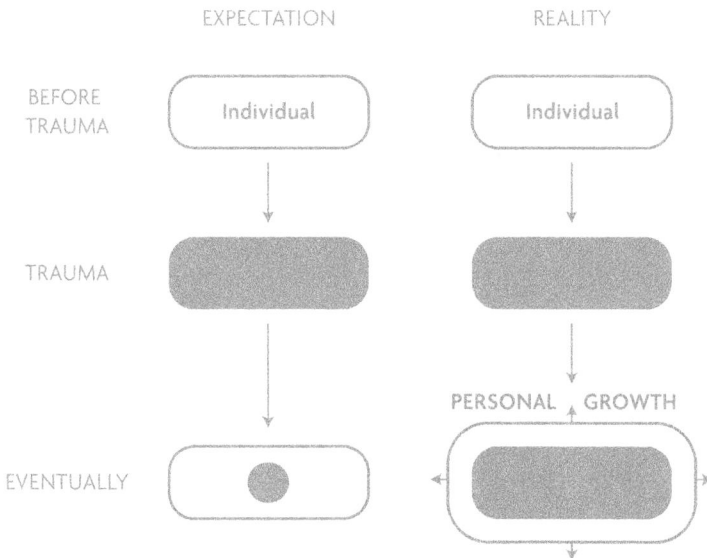

In sum, these findings suggest that there is a clinical advantage in identifying, focusing on and building people's strengths to help them cope with difficult experiences, as opposed to purely focusing on reducing negative emotions and stresses. Rather than solely trying to eliminate negative experiences (moving from –5 to 0 in Fig. 1), it is also essential to help facilitate coping skills and utilise people's strengths to promote wellbeing (moving towards +5). Irrespective of the level of stress, accessing our personal resources and strengths is most important if we are to maintain psychological wellbeing.

In naturopathic practice, my approach to helping people with health issues is always to capitalise on their constitutional strengths and resources, while also drawing upon nature (through natural remedies and strategies) to expedite the natural and innate self-recuperative powers that exist within us all.

Misconception #3: If you correct your weaknesses, you will perform at your optimum

Many teachers, employers, parents, and leaders believe that optimal performance results from fixing weaknesses. To promote professional development, employees are typically exposed to training programs that zero in on deficits. Evaluation interviews often focus on areas that need improvement and aspects of work that employees are struggling with. Many schools have taken a similar approach for decades. (It was the case when I was at school so that's a long time indeed!) Typically, the number of mistakes is highlighted when work is corrected and when report cards are brought home, and lower grades tend to attract more attention. But does correcting weakness result in an optimally functioning person or organisation? Fixing weakness alone will at best help the individual or organisation to become 'normal' but may also be a recipe for mediocrity. This is analogous to reaching 0 on the scale in Fig. 1, which is not the same as getting to +5.

FET and meditation for developing potential

Flower essence therapy gives equal weight to positive potentials as to negative qualities when choosing an appropriate flower essence, as we have seen in examples such as St John's Wort and Pink Yarrow flower essences discussed earlier. In meditation, rather than focusing on suppressing or eliminating negative thoughts and feelings, a level of acceptance is reached so that, though they remain present, they do not have their previous negative impact.

Research findings show that the opportunity to do what one does best each day (that is, using one's strengths) is a core predictor of workplace engagement and performance (Harter et al., 2003). This approach is often taken in elite sport. I recall the captain of a successful Australian cricket team saying in response to a question about the improvement seen in certain members of the team: 'We have allowed those players the freedom to go out and play *their* game. Play to their strengths and the rest will take care of itself. … Sure there were a couple of tweaks made to some minor weaknesses in their technique, but the main change was giving them permission to play *their* [best] way.' Boosting awareness and using strengths, rather than just removing weaknesses, will contribute to optimal performance (analogous to getting to +5 on the Fig. 1 scale).

Misconception #4: If you focus on your weaknesses, your strengths will take care of themselves

Another misconception that contributes to an excessive focus on weakness involves the belief that strengths do not need much attention because they will take care of themselves and develop naturally. However, people often need to be made aware of the strengths they possess, for instance by reminding them of how they have successfully navigated and managed a difficult situation in the past. Just like skills, strengths can be trained and developed deliberately. For example, research has shown that, through practice, people can learn to be more optimistic (Meevissen et al., 2011). Boosting strengths through practice and effort increases frequency of use, but also a person learns to apply her/his strengths in more and different situations. While a person remains unaware of their strengths, they won't practise using them or learn how to best utilise them, and so their potential to improve their sense of wellbeing is not realised. When a very creative child is not exposed to activities that call upon creativity, the child is unlikely to develop skills, knowledge, and experience that will maximise their creative potential. Although many strengths are already present at a very young age, they need to be recognised and nurtured to realise their full potential.

I found that this was also the case with some young and inexperienced students I taught at a Melbourne naturopathic college some years ago. A common question from younger students who had commenced the course straight out of Secondary School was, 'How will I develop rapport, or get my clients to have faith in me and my advice, when I have so little life experience?' One young woman asked: 'How can I give health and lifestyle advice to a menopausal woman, or harder still, a mid-life male?' I replied that the most important thing is a strong desire to develop rapport, and if they simply be themselves, a good connection is likely to grow. If a student remains focused on their inadequacies, they will never even make a start! Once they take the plunge with the right intention and act with good will, they will realise that they already have some social skills they can put to good use.

FET, meditation, and recognising your strengths

A correctly chosen flower essence will help you to bring your own strengths into awareness and enhance them. The qualities you look for in an individual to prescribe their appropriate flower essence include both weaknesses and potential strengths. Once again, St John's Wort and Pink Yarrow flower essences are good examples.

It is interesting also to note that children learn meditation easily because most of them haven't as yet lost touch with what is a natural and innate ability to experience a deeply relaxed state of mind. Just as an injured limb will eventually suffer from atrophy from extended lack of use, so too can the ability to achieve a natural and deeply relaxed state be almost lost through lack of experience by those growing up in an 'external to self'-focused, fast and over-stimulating world. As adults, we need to regularly practise meditation, to re-visit, engage and fully experience this completely natural and innate strength that human beings possess.

Misconception #5: If you focus on your weaknesses, you will prevent problems in the future

There is no doubt that a focus on repairing weakness will discover ways to decrease the gap between –5 and 0 (Fig. 1). It is important to have different interventions and treatment programs to deal with problems and setbacks. However, the disease model has not moved us much closer to the *prevention* of health problems, and in the majority of cases, even when it assists in recovery and helps to manage a health problem or slow its progress, it does not cure it or prevent a relapse. Most therapeutic interventions are primarily aimed at fixing health issues after they have already developed, rather than preventing them from arising in the first place. When it comes to prevention, the question is not: 'How can we treat people with problem X effectively?' but 'How can problem X be prevented from occurring or re-occurring?' How can we prevent serious problems like burnout, depression, substance abuse or other mental and physical diseases from becoming chronic?

For example, our main approach to pandemics is retrospective in the sense that currently, medical science's greatest tool against the spread of disease is the development of vaccines. Unfortunately, this will always be like shutting the door after the horse has bolted; great damage has already been done before a vaccine can be produced and disseminated. If we ask instead: 'How can our susceptibility to a potentially virulent virus be prevented in future?' we might come up with a useful response such as, 'Let's build on our strengths and innate healing potential, focusing on how we maintain and enhance our natural immunity NOW, to protect against ALL types of pathogens, including ones we haven't yet encountered.' As we have seen, Positive Psychology research asserts that it is not the absence or avoidance of stresses—viruses in this case—but rather utilisation of strengths and resources that gives us the *ability to effectively deal with all types of stresses (including viruses).*

I believe major advances in prevention can occur when we build competency rather than just correct weakness. To design effective prevention programs, we must also focus on the 0 to +5 range and ask: 'Why do some people display resilience and flourish despite difficult circumstances?' and 'What are the characteristics of these resilient and flourishing individuals, and what can we learn from them?'

With regard to our physical health we might ask: 'What are the characteristics, individual constitutions, lifestyle behaviours and health approaches of people who display strong immunity and natural resilience/recovery from ailments, and/or maintain a level of health and wellbeing that doesn't devolve into chronic disease?' If we look again at the example of a pandemic, it is important to establish an understanding of who the most vulnerable in our communities are, and take measures to protect them. But it is even more important, I believe, to investigate and understand those who are *best* equipped in their natural ability to display strong immunity and resilience when exposed or infected and learn from them.

We need to find natural approaches and medicines that potentiate, maintain, and safeguard our own innate natural immunity and healing responses to all diseases. Therapies that take a holistic view can inform us greatly about answers in this respect. These types of therapies, including FET and meditation, examine people's strengths and vulnerabilities and tap into their existing internal and external resources. We need to learn how to use this knowledge to design interventions that help people to cope better and display resilience when life gets tough, OR remain healthy despite the threat of exposure to external pathogens.

A WELLNESS MODEL OF HEALTH

Since beginning his work in this area in 1998, Martin Seligman has encouraged the field of psychology to expand its scope beyond problems and pathology to include human flourishing. According to Seligman (2002), positive psychology aims to move people not from −5 to 0 but from 0 to +5 (see Fig. 1), and to do this, a change of focus is needed from what is wrong with people to *what is right with people*, and towards learning how to boost their strengths.

The questions that positive psychology aims to answer are: What characteristics do people with high levels of happiness possess? What qualities do people who manage their troubles effectively have? What are their strengths? These questions do not fit within the disease model. In shifting our enquiry towards what is right with people, we move to a *wellness* model of health. As it happens, this has been the obsession of naturopathy since its beginnings as the Nature Cure in the nineteenth century! The naturopathic approach is based on the premise that every individual possesses an innate self-recuperative power, a natural resilience that is nature-driven. Naturopaths assist an individual to tap into what is already there, what is already RIGHT within them! More than right, Mother Nature is perfect and always finds a way!! Naturopaths (and other natural therapists such as practitioners of Traditional Chinese Medicine, Homeopathy, and Ayurvedic Medicine) use natural medicines and natural methods to support this innate self-recuperative power. If we learn what differentiates naturally happy and resilient people from unhappy and non-resilient people, we can use this knowledge to increase happiness and boost the resilience of those for whom wellness doesn't come so naturally.

When naturopaths take a client's health history, they are looking to find out what level of wellbeing the client already has, what health-inducing dietary, exercise and relaxation practices they already engage in, how often they get sick, and what type of illnesses they tend to get—and most importantly, how well do they recover from illness and show resilience afterwards? These questions and others inform us about someone's current general health—their susceptibility to disease and degree of potential for recovery, irrespective of whether or not they currently have any symptoms of illness. So an important aspect of positive psychology research is to investigate human behaviour using a *strengths* approach, with a focus on human flourishing and markers of psychological wellbeing that characterises the wellness model. A naturopath's role is *NOT ONLY to identify vulnerabilities* and potential for illness but *ALSO to identify strengths and natural resources already available*. Iridology is one of the diagnostic tools I use which is able to identify both general vulnerabilities and constitutional strengths. Natural remedies such as flower essences are prescribed on the basis of this information, taking into account both negative or maladaptive tendencies and positive, adaptive strengths.

By merely correcting weakness—the disease model of health— we will not create optimal performance or wellbeing. However, it is also true that only focusing on strengths—the wellness model—while ignoring weaknesses will not automatically lead to optimal performance or wellbeing either. When weaknesses cause problems or hinder optimal capacity for health, they need to be addressed and managed. While some traditional psychologists may believe that taking away negatives will automatically create positives, positive psychologists and many natural health practitioners avoid the trap of believing that creating positives will automatically take away the negatives. Attention must be paid to processes for building the positive and to processes for coping with and recovering from the negative. Naturopaths pay attention to natural strategies/treatments that build and maintain overall health and wellbeing—*remaining disease-free*—as well as paying attention to natural strategies/treatments that address a current disease—and aid *becoming disease-free*.

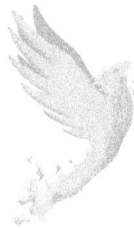

EMOTIONAL AWARENESS

We have already spoken about how, whenever we try to repress a natural human experience—whether it be our hunger, thirst, pain, fatigue, or emotions—we can only do so successfully for a limited time. The energy required for repression means that our conscious self-regulatory resources become exhausted, and our innate need grows strong enough to overpower them.

REASONS *NOT* TO AVOID OR SUPPRESS EMOTION

1. It is not healthy in the long run

An analogy I often use is that supressing emotion is like trying to hold a beach ball underwater. Since this goes against the beach ball's natural state, it takes considerable effort to hold it under, and even with effort, it will only stay submerged for so long before it bounces back to the surface. Furthermore, the deeper we push it down, the greater the struggle to hold it there, and the more force the ball will have when it reemerges, *erupting* out of the water. This is similar to our emotions— we may suppress them for a time, but when they reemerge, they are even *stronger* than before, and ironically, they may *erupt* over something seemingly trivial and unrelated to the event that caused them in the first place. Try as we might, we cannot keep our emotions repressed forever, as it is mentally and physically exhausting, often resulting in physical illness and the failure of our natural immunity.

A hyper-emotional release is small compensation for our efforts during those times when we don't respond, as the reaction is so disproportionate to the incident that no one takes our 'eruption' seriously. Those around respond by either ignoring it or dismissing it. Despite the fact that the original trauma was real and has led to a build-up of valid emotional tension, people still respond with: 'There he goes again, the angry so and so!' or worse, 'Oh, she's flying off again, it must be that time of the month.' No one takes your reaction seriously even though there is strong justification for it. You feel as though you are not heard and consequently become frustrated beyond reason; you retreat emotionally and the vicious cycle continues. The most tragic aspect of this pattern is that we may deny ourselves the opportunity to explore and understand 'core emotions ... such as grief, deep seated anger or rejection' (FES; Wells, *Essential Flower Essence Book* p. 185).

FET and meditation for release of suppressed emotions

Fuchsia flower essence, which we discussed earlier in relation to secondary, reactive emotions, is a great help for people stuck in a vicious cycle of supressing or under-reacting to their emotional responses, only to have them erupt later in an over-reaction to a minor incident, or manifest in the form of illness. Fuchsia helps break this cycle, providing an inner freedom to make emotional choices from a position of greater awareness, especially in the moment. This deeper awareness and self-understanding results in genuine emotional expression.

One of the benefits of regular meditation practice is that you are more *grounded* in the moment and accepting of your genuine, primary emotional responses. Mindful awareness also gives you more choices about what you express and how you act on primary responses.

2. Your body keeps a record of emotional events

The poet Maya Angelou is often quoted as saying, 'I've learned that people will forget what you said, people will forget what you did, but people will never forget how you made them feel.' Emotions, especially strong ones such as those associated with trauma, 'live on' in the body. In *The Body Keeps the Score* (2015), psychiatrist Dr Bessel van der Kolk describes how trauma impacts our physicality. Specifically, he shows that individuals who experience trauma are more likely to experience physical symptoms later in life, including diabetes, autoimmune disorders, and heart disease. If painful emotions are repressed instead of processed with some level of awareness, this can lead to negative physical outcomes. Here is an example from my clinical practice.

Case study: Coming to maturity

In her early teens, 'Jane' was brought to me for a consultation by her mother, who explained that their home environment was difficult, and that Jane had been facing significant challenges. Jane's father had experienced a mental health episode a year earlier, which was compounded by self-medicating with alcohol. He had become very aggressive and intimidating towards Jane on a number of occasions. Understandably, this was very traumatic for her, as the younger and more vulnerable of two siblings. Though the father was now in better mental health, things at home were still far from good and the relationship between father and both daughters was strained. Jane had developed alopecia in the last couple of months—a distressing hair-loss condition that has the potential to become chronic—and had become lethargic and lost a lot of motivation, very unlike how she had been before. She had become closed and didn't want to talk about things with her mother anymore. I prescribed the following flower essences.

Flower essence for restored trust: Hibiscus (FES group)

Jane had experienced extreme emotional hurt and loss of trust.

Negative state
Guarded, often due to past emotional abuse or harsh treatment (FES)
Closed mind; 'lack of warmth and vitality' (FES)

Positive state
Regained trust
Open-minded, warm and receptive
(Wells, *Essential Flower Essence Book* p. 204)

Flower essence for renewed interest in life: Wild Rose (Bach group)

Jane was experiencing apathy, exhaustion and low vitality as a consequence of feeling let down.

Negative state
Withdrawn resignation
Disinterested and dispirited

Positive state
Enthusiastic and involved
Renewed interest and passion for life
(Wells, *Essential Flower Essence Book* p. 368)

Internalisation of strong emotion through suppression requires enormous conscious (and unconscious) self-regulatory resources that ultimately become exhausted, as we have described earlier. According to naturopathic philosophy, this lowering of vitality makes a person more susceptible to acute illness in the form of shallow, short-lived health crises. If these attempts by the body to restore balance/homeostasis are not treated naturally (or if acute episodes don't occur at all), deeper and potentially more chronic health issues may develop. Although Jane had been more nervous and apprehensive at home after her father's outbursts, she hadn't had any colds or other acute ailments, but had eventually developed the more deep-seated condition of alopecia. (This was a very different pattern from her older sister who, 'as soon as she got rid of one cold would get another,' according to her mother.)

Dr van der Kolk's research showed how trauma can later find expression through chronic physical ailments. His research findings are consistent with naturopathic philosophy, and, as one Traditional Chinese Therapy practitioner said to me: 'The body often expresses what people find it difficult to say.' Jane's alopecia was ultimately cured when she was able to process deep emotions that she, understandably, had had difficulty in expressing. This was facilitated and supported by counselling sessions and the prescribed flower essences.

3. What you resist will persist!

Sleepless Dogs
Something remained after the exchange—
A bit of hurt, a bit of anger, a bit of not-sure-what.
I thought it through (I thought)
But more came later, tied in a hopeless knot.

What is it with feelings that can't be thought out?
Stuff that stays and eats away
From outside in
And all the way into the next day,
And the next, and the next …

Only one way to unravel the snarl thus sewn:
Go back and engage the seamster.
With caution, awaken this sleeper—
Untangle the unsaid words
And make them your own.

Repressing emotions only gives them more energy, as I depicted using the analogy of the beachball—you can only hold it under the surface for so long before you tire and the ball erupts out of the water. Also, if we manage to keep emotions repressed and 'under wraps' long enough, they become less and less familiar to us, as many people experience when they come off antidepressants too quickly and without sufficient support. In a research article titled 'Antidepressant Withdrawal and Rebound Phenomena' (2019), Henssler et al. found that many people suffered severe relapses into depression after discontinuing antidepressants because re-experiencing emotions that have become unfamiliar often makes them feel scarier and more overwhelming than before. This is especially true if we were taking antidepressants in the first place because of difficulty in managing and knowing how to respond to emotions.

Meditation and flower essences for facing intense emotions

The practice of meditation involves NOT resisting or suppressing emotions, even when they previously had a negative effect and felt uncomfortable. Emotion is allowed to remain present, while we are in an overall state of *calm, natural ease and stillness*. We establish a different relationship with our feelings, and can come to accept them in a way that ultimately reduces their negative impact. What you don't resist may still persist, but it becomes less and less of a demon. Feelings are present but we are able to understand that they are not all we are—we are much more! Then emotions can become just a great source of information and feedback about the environment and how to respond to it in the most appropriate manner.

Flower essences are a key element of my practice when supporting someone coming off antidepressants—a process that is carried out under the supervision of a medical doctor. Flower essences not only help a person navigate the issues associated with their initial withdrawal from a drug (Antidepressant Discontinuation Syndrome) but also enable them to commence working with the issues that created the need for antidepressants in the first place. The most appropriate flower essences are different for each individual and change throughout the process.

4. When you disconnect from your emotions you disconnect from your authentic Self

An important aspect of authenticity is being in connection in the moment, with our own emotional experience. If not, we behave in a disingenuous way with our Self and others. Knowing what we are feeling, and the purpose and reasons for our feelings, and how to communicate these feelings—all this is part of being in touch with and expressing our authentic Self. Repressing our primary emotions is essentially ignoring who we are, and this causes stress when there is conflict between the urge for authentic Self-expression and the anxiety-driven wish to maintain and present an inauthentic persona to the world. Conversely, when we allow ourselves to feel and respond to our primary emotions, we know and understand ourselves better by staying connected with the essential part of our being which is our authentic Self. All flower essences help us to (re-)connect with some aspect of our true Self.

Flower essence for authentic Self-expression: Goldenrod (FES group)

A flower essence that is especially helpful in this process of authentic Self-expression is Goldenrod, which 'encourages us to be unambiguous and *genuine in our intentions and the expression of our feelings,* and stops us being easily distracted from our truth by external social pressures' (Wells, *Essential Flower Essence Book* p. 193). The plant's Latin name *Solidago* (from *solidus*, meaning *whole*) indicates its use as a physical wound-healing herb. The flower essence, working on a deeper dynamic level, helps heal emotional wounds so that we can feel and integrate all aspects of the Self. We become *whole* again, enabling the true and *authentic* Self to be expressed. Unresolved emotional wounds cause us to act in a less-than-integrated way and make us more inclined to express a false or negative persona to the world. Goldenrod helps us to feel more relaxed about ourselves and remain true to our higher Self, especially around other people.

Negative state
Too easily influenced by family, peers and social groups (FES)
Inauthentic and unable to be true to oneself
Unable to adhere to inner conviction

Positive state
Comfortable in your skin; authentic
Well-developed individuality [along with] social consciousness (FES)
(Wells, *Essential Flower Essence Book* p. 193)

When we practise meditation, we pause to reconnect with our inner Self, associated with *calm, natural ease and stillness* within. Dr Rudolf Steiner spoke of this inner resource as the authentic *I*, and Carl Jung spoke of it in terms of the *Self* as distinct from the *persona*; other therapists simply speak of the *true self*.

5. Emotions are a necessary part of being human

Emotions are a vital element of living. It is impossible to go through life without experiencing a vast array of emotions. However, when we are in the habit of *repressing* and/or *avoiding* our more difficult emotions, this also robs us of our ability to truly feel our more positive/joyful ones.

Repressing emotion robs us of our chance to be fully alive:
'Real liberation comes not from glossing over or repressing painful states of feeling, but only from experiencing them to the full.'
(Carl Jung)

Avoiding emotion means we're only half alive:
'Tis better to have loved and lost than never to have loved at all.'
(Alfred Tennyson)

Sometimes you have to risk feeling difficult emotions in order to experience joyful ones! Or as Carl Jung says, 'we have to risk life to get into life, then it takes on colour, otherwise we might as well read a book' (quoted in Dunne, 2015 p. 114). When we share our emotional experiences we connect with other individuals on a deeper and more intimate level. Relationships are built upon sharing vulnerable moments, which require us to 'feel together.' A life without emotions would be a very shallow and lonely experience indeed! Nevertheless, people are often reluctant or even ashamed to share their feelings. In this situation, Pink Monkeyflower flower essence can help.

Flower essence for emotional courage: Pink Monkeyflower (FES group)

This flower essence allows a person to display 'emotional transparency [and have the] courage to take emotional risks with others' (FES). Like all of the Monkeyflower flower essences, Pink Monkeyflower helps people raise their awareness of certain intense emotions that they may fear and/or feel uncomfortable expressing and can help a person overcome a self-denigrating sense of shame and unworthiness about the feelings they wish to express (Wells, *Essential Flower Essence Book* p. 398).

Mindfulness is a product of regular meditation that can enable us to reach a level of acceptance of our emotions and feelings, allowing them to be fully present and have full rein if we desire. We feel the freedom that comes from experiencing them so that we live life to the full!

REPRESSED EMOTION IN PHYSICAL ILLNESS

'To cherish secrets and hold back emotion is a psychic misdemeanour for which nature finally visits us with sickness.'
(Carl Jung, *Collected Works*)

In her book, *Chiron and the Healing Journey* (2009), Melanie Reinhart states: '[S]uffering is present in everyone's life but relating with wisdom and compassion to our own experience turns "poison into medicine."' She encourages us to consider the degree to which we engage with our dis-ease or illness—whether we choose to fully experience it or attempt to suppress it. Pharmaceutical drugs may play an important and humane role in temporarily ameliorating our uncomfortable physical symptoms and/or helping us to manage them, but in doing so they also can prevent the physical body's full expression of disease that emerges from much deeper in our being. This can obscure the potential to gain understanding, insight and wisdom by discovering the root causes of our disease or illness.

Health approaches that recognise and seek to understand the natural wisdom behind physical and disease symptoms as well as manage them, are crucial for young children, who are still in the process of developing. My many years of experience have enabled me to observe and follow health patterns across the generations in families. Part of Rudolf Steiner's philosophy (the basis for Anthroposophical Medicine) is that the first seven years of life are profoundly important and also provide a great opportunity to change the direction of generational health for the better, influencing inherited issues in a positive way. A naturopathic approach to children's health, safely brings relief from illness, and guides and supports wellness, providing a real opportunity to resolve deeper, inherited, constitutional health weaknesses and vulnerabilities.

I'm not suggesting here that we put up with truly painful symptoms, and of course we must take immediate medical action in potentially serious situations! I am advocating that we might make more effort to utilise natural approaches where possible and learn to perceive the deeper causes and meanings behind the symptoms of disease.

Flower essences and meditation support natural healing

Natural remedies such as flower essences, herbal remedies, and homeopathic medicines don't suppress symptoms. They do help to ameliorate and ease them while enabling the body (and mind) to bring about an efficient and natural resolution of illness. In meditation, when we experience difficult emotions and allow them to pass, we come to accept them and they lose their power over us, as described earlier in relation to chronic pain. Paradoxically, if we can learn to relax and be less resistant and fearful of discomfort (while seeking advice from qualified health professionals), the body and mind can get on with the job of healing more quickly and easily. What you resist persists, and what you don't resist, desists!

In my naturopathic practice, I have often noticed that, as natural treatment progresses, clients forget many of the symptoms they had been suffering from—not because they are suppressed and 'out of sight, out of mind,' but because they have been properly processed and are now 'out of mind, out of sight.' My experience with migraine headaches provides a practical example I will describe in more detail later, but, briefly, as a young man I suffered from debilitating migraines. They regularly laid me out flat until I realised that my body and mind wanted rest and time out, and if I didn't let that happen voluntarily, well, it would happen involuntarily! Fully engaging with my disease at its deeper roots ultimately helped me to become free of migraines.

When you can view any significant illness or your particular 'wound' as having purpose and meaning, you give yourself a powerful tool to assist recovery—your 'wound' becomes a source of healing and insight. In my case it allowed me to become what Jung called a 'wounded healer.' Remain open and receptive to the profound insights being conveyed to you by your body—it is always telling you something. Be receptive to the message in the body because its 'woundedness,' its posture and even its shape are outer expressions of your innermost thoughts, feelings and beliefs. The state of the body's health can provide insights from the subconscious, where our Self-concept dwells. As Jung put it, the body and psyche are two sides of the same coin. They are inseparable.

As part of a healing process, emotions/feelings that we may find difficult to acknowledge, experience fully and therefore process, often 'work their way out' from deeper levels of our being in the psyche and manifest as physical illness.

Displacement of emotional trauma: Our 'message in a body'

As a natural therapist, I often see people whose anxiety and emotional distress has been ameliorated by the onset of a skin eruption, a head cold, a migraine, loose bowel motions etc. Then the job of the healer is to ameliorate the discomfort of these more superficial/acute symptoms, rather than suppress them, and thus allow them to quickly resolve in the way the body's natural recuperative processes intended. If emotions are suppressed 'successfully' this process of displacing emotional trauma onto the body can occur in a short period after the initial trauma occurs, but the displacement can also take years. We have mentioned previously how psychiatrist Bessel van der Kolk's research showed that unresolved trauma impacts our physicality. Specifically, he found that individuals who experience trauma are more likely to exhibit physical conditions later in life such as diabetes, autoimmune disorders, and heart disease. If emotions associated with trauma are suppressed instead of processed with some level of awareness, the likelihood that there will be negative physical repercussions is high.

Scientific research, especially in the area of psychoneuroimmunology, provides much evidence that emotions and attitudes have a significant effect on our physical health. Depression and long-term emotional stress causes the release of cortisol, and this suppresses the immune system, which is responsible for our natural defences against illness. It has been shown, for example, that when a partner in a long-standing relationship dies, the incidence of the surviving partner becoming seriously ill within the next 18 months is far greater than normal. The traumatic impact of unresolved emotions associated with grief eventually manifests as disease on the physical level.

At some time in our lives, most of us have been living proof of the connection between the experience of prolonged stress and illness, whether that illness manifests as a head cold or something more severe. Our cognitive emotional self-regulatory resources eventually become depleted, our overall vitality declines and our natural immune system fails us. If we listen to the body, and receive its message loud and clear that we need to rest and allow healing to occur, we can identify and manage our emotional stresses better—and when we do this we usually recover well.

Emotional messages expressed through the body can be heard, and their meaning understood if we choose to listen closely (with the support of qualified medical practitioners). We can identify the *implicate*—the psyche's message—in the *explicate*—the physical body's disease symptoms. In this section, I will provide a few specific examples of physical ailments and elaborate on their psychological implications. In doing this I am drawing on forty years of experience in practice as a naturopath and counsellor, but also on current body-mind research, psychoneuroimmunology, traditional knowledge, anthroposophical medicine, esoteric literature, and common *sense*.

In his essay 'Spirit and Life,' Carl Jung asserts: '[M]ind and body are the expression of a single entity.' In traditional Chinese medicine (TCM), emotions and physical health are also understood as intimately connected. An integrated mind-body approach to health and healing, as in TCM, operates in a dynamic loop where emotions impact the health of the body and vice versa.

Figure 3. How emotions and organs are connected in TCM

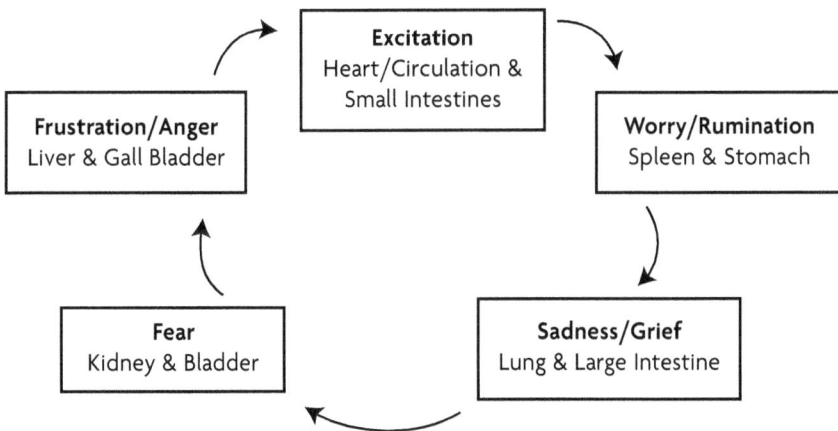

Because illness is an external consequence of a person's unique process occurring deep within their being, rather than a random, senseless event, we have a *choice* about how we respond to it. We can *choose* to reflect on our illness and perceive meaning. Over the years I have worked with thousands of clients who have gained insight into their illnesses to enable them to become healthier.

'MESSAGES IN THE BODY': EXAMPLES

Stress responses

When life is physically threatened, the adrenal glands on top of the kidneys release the fast-acting stress hormone adrenalin into the bloodstream. This makes more blood available to muscle tissues of the limbs to prepare for fight or flight (although in some cases there can be a 'freeze' response also). This 'fear, fight, or flight' mechanism can save our life when we are physically challenged or under threat. Adrenalin injections are used as a last-ditch effort to save life in some cases of collapse. Cortisol, a slower-acting stress hormone also secreted by the adrenals is likewise produced in response to threat, and works to suppress non-essential functions during a crisis and help the body recover afterwards. It is used in the treatment of life-threatening conditions such as extreme (anaphylactic) allergic reactions and asthma.

Unfortunately, many people today suffer from *stress syndrome* in which these hormones, and especially cortisol, are produced continually in response to multiple stressors. Even if none of these stressors are life-threatening, the adrenal glands remain in a constant state of overstimulation and overactivity, often associated with high blood pressure. Unresolved emotional trauma can also induce this state as we have seen previously.

People suffering from stress syndrome may feel restless, with a strong sense of urgency—too much to do and too little time to do it in—and live in a constant state of anxious agitation. The stimulated adrenals have them ready for action but because there is no single life-threatening emergency to respond to, they often feel 'driven with nowhere to drive.' If they are unable to manage their stress levels, eventually they become adrenally fatigued to the point of exhaustion and burnout (see Olive flower essence below). The message from the body here is to learn how to manage unavoidable stresses better and avoid unnecessary stress by making lifestyle adjustments.

Meditation and flower essences for stress syndrome

There is no better single response after getting this stress syndrome message from the body than to start practising meditation. Many research findings show that meditation helps us to manage our reactions to stress better, significantly lessening negative health impacts. Regularly feeling *calm, natural ease and stillness* during meditation helps you 'reboot' each time you practise but also increasingly allows *calmness* to infiltrate the rest of your day. This facilitates quicker recovery from burnout and lessens the likelihood of relapse. Energy and vitality are restored and conserved. FET is also a proactive response to hearing the body's message. Olive flower essence is one of many to consider.

Flower essence for recovery from exhaustion: Olive (Bach group)

The olive tree continues to flower and bear fruit generation after generation, conserving and maintaining its reserves of energy even into advanced old age. This capacity is represented by the storage of concentrated oils in the dense fruit. Olive fruit is the plant's focal point, packed full of complex nutrient substances, making it a dynamic and compact natural food supplement (Wells, *Essential Flower Essence Book* p. 261). When cut back to a stump, new stems emerge from the wood of even the oldest olive trees—natural resilience is displayed overtly in all aspects of the plant.

Negative state
Too tired to complete tasks
Exhausted on all levels

Positive state
Capable of sustained, dynamically applied effort
Re-vitalised and peaceful

Female health

Metaphysically, the uterus represents the feminine principle, and is regarded as the seat of creativity for a woman. On a physical level this can be seen in the way the uterus provides an environment that nurtures the growth of a human being, expressing creativity in the form of procreation. During each menstrual cycle the uterus prepares to receive a fertilised ovum and nurture and nourish the growth of the foetus. Physical health problems affecting the female reproductive organs may relate to difficulty in finding creative expression in other areas of life. Are you able to fully nurture and bring to fruition your own creativity? Does your life support the initiation, nurturing and expression of thoughts and ideas you feel passionate about, or do you feel inhibited or restricted in these areas? Do you feel stifled in your ability to emotionally and creatively express yourself day to day and in your life in general? One significant issue that many women have had to negotiate throughout history and into the present has been the difficulty of balancing procreative expression—having children—with creative expression in other areas of their lives. Pressures regarding women's stereotypical cultural roles within a patriarchal society have had a repressive influence on many lives. A choice to engage fully in creative expression outside the family has too often been denied. Fortunately, things are changing for the better, though too slowly for many. Pomegranate flower essence directly addresses the issue of finding creative balance between family and career, and feminine and masculine sides, for both sexes.

Flower essence for creative expression: Pomegranate (FES group)

Traditionally, pomegranate fruits have been seen as a symbol of fertility and creativity because they are thought to resemble the uterus, and the rich red colour of flowers and fruits symbolises the life-giving blood that flows to it. In Greek mythology the goddess Hera is sometimes depicted holding a pomegranate, with its red fruit full of seeds representing femininity and womanhood. Pomegranate flower essence relates to the capacity for creative expression, especially for women.

What makes Pomegranate flower essence especially relevant today— and why I have prescribed it often in my practice—is its ability to help when there is a need for separation and balance between potentially conflicting roles. For example, parents, and stereotypically especially mothers, need to constantly 'put on different hats,' compartmentalising life as they move between roles of nurturing at home and career people out in the world. Kaminski and Katz (FES) tell us that Pomegranate flower essence can help to achieve creative balance between procreation and creativity, and between family and career (Wells, *Essential Flower Essence Book* pp. 277–78).

Negative state
Emotionally exclusive; divided allegiances
Confusion over family/career balance (FES)

Positive state
Emotionally inclusive; embracing all aspects of life
Clear, creative direction in life (FES)

Case study: The menstrual cycle

For my client 'Jenny,' problems associated with her menstrual cycle were a reflection of an inner struggle for acceptance of her feminine side—what Jung called the *anima*. Rejection, denial or resistance to the feminine aspects of the psyche may manifest in problems in the female reproductive organs. Jane was, in her own words, 'high achieving and highly driven,' and was running her own very successful business with a number of happy and loyal employees. She consulted me at my clinic for significant PMS and severe menstrual pain of long standing. During the session she explained that she 'resented that time of the month with a passion,' believing it responsible for making her feel 'out of it' and unable to function at her best. She suffered silently, keeping to herself many quite severe menstrual symptoms and would 'fight them—not give in to them, or just dope myself up with painkillers to get through the day.' I believe that raising awareness of aspects of self and psyche that are implicate in physical ailments—which may themselves be denied, resisted or suppressed—creates opportunities for personal growth and ultimately better health. Jenny, to her credit, was very interested in 'achieving' both personal growth and better health! Strong and determined, just prior to coming to see me she had fortuitously done some real soul searching and said: 'The main reason I push myself so hard, I reckon, is because I'm trying to prove something, and probably to my dad. He's never given me credit for anything.' Based on this and other indications, I prescribed Sunflower flower essence (and a couple of other natural medicines to help purely on the physical level.)

A few days after the consultation, she called me and explained how, in the middle of a working day, she had pulled over into a bayside car park and was gazing out over the water. This type of time out was unheard of for her! She opened the conversation with, 'What the hell have you put in those drops? I can't be bothered doing anything today!' I asked her if everything was under control at work and she replied, 'Yes everything is fine but I never take time out like this on a working day. Amazingly, I don't give a stuff—and I haven't even got my period!' Long story short, this was the beginning of a change of attitude to her work and life. The following day she got back to work as usual but her priorities had already shifted slightly, and one change was to give herself much more 'me time' as she put it—'once I got to know what that actually was!' She became kinder to herself—more nurturing—and acknowledged some needs she had been denying 'just to prove something to someone else.' She began to feel less resistance to the arrival of her period, taking a little time out and lowering her workload for a day or two, 'because I can!'

After a few months, 'that time of month' had become significantly less uncomfortable, and fewer and fewer painkillers were required. Applying a Jungian perspective to this transformation, we can see that Jenny had eventually come to a place of far greater acceptance of the part of her that is uniquely and overtly female and which, yes, may leave her feeling slightly more vulnerable (rather than 'sooky' as she once described herself) for a short while. Her unconscious male side—the Jungian *animus* principle, heavily influenced by her father's biases in her formative years—had showed little tolerance or understanding of what she had learnt to view as female 'weaknesses.' From what Jenny said, I gathered that her father was definitely not in touch with his feminine side! Taking Sunflower flower essence enabled her to make some subtle but positive and profound shifts within her psyche's masculine side so that she was more able to embrace her feminine side. Over time, she was able to be more herself, more true to her inner authority and her own personal values, without the need to conform to anyone else's value system—especially her father's.

According to Jung the growth and development of the anima involves opening up to *emotionality*—a paradigm shift in consciousness that involves intuitive responsiveness, creativity and imagination, and *greater psychological sensitivity towards oneself and others.*

Flower essence for Self-authority: Sunflower (FES group)

Negative state
Poor relationship to authority and/or father
Self-inflation or self-effacement (FES) or vacillating between the two

Positive state
Aligned with your inner (higher) authority
Upstanding, honourable and 'your own person'
(Wells, *Essential Flower Essence Book* p. 330)

Case study: Fertility

If a woman wants to have a child and is having trouble conceiving when there are no physiological impediments, there may be issues of receptivity on deeper levels. There are obviously many things that influence this—her relationship with her partner; stress and the rapid pace of life; her ability to find relaxation and ease. (Of course, all this equally applies to her partner or whoever is emotionally close to her.)

For my client 'Kate,' participation in an IVF program meant that intimate encounters had become clinical and lacking the spontaneity that allows a woman (and her partner) to relax and be deeply receptive. Kate and her husband had been trying to conceive for the best part of a year. Kate was a very capable person, a well-respected teacher, reliable, knowledgeable, fit and healthy, and seemingly able to do anything she put her mind to. She had always been able to achieve her goals with, as she put it, 'a plan of action and hard work.' But, alas, her plan of action had failed this time. All relevant medical tests were clear, she was on the best diet, she was taking the recommended natural supplements to support reproductive health, and she was also acutely aware of her cycle and the times she would be most likely to conceive. Her husband, with whom she had a strong and supportive relationship, joked that he was just the sperm donor part of her program. Kate had a definite and very well-informed plan that didn't seem to be working out.

I prescribed what I believed was the most appropriate flower essence, Impatiens, as it fitted well with her state of mind and predicament. I prescribed little else as she had most things covered! We also had a chat about the need for spontaneity and time out just to chill and smell the roses, because a plan that was too rigid might work against what she was trying to achieve—a relaxed and receptive state of mind and body.

Kate came back to see me three weeks later and, not surprisingly, she had taken her drops religiously! There was a definite shift in her perspective and demeanour. A big part of it was that she had reached a point where she accepted that there might have to be a 'Plan B' if she didn't conceive in the near future. This was a revolutionary change for Kate, as Plan A had always worked for her in the past! Plan B was that she would reconsider her career opportunities and follow other interests and activities that she and her husband wanted to try. In other words, she would spend more time enjoying herself, accepting and being open to whatever else might happen! She continued taking her flower essence over the next month and returned to see me around 6 weeks after we had begun working together. At this meeting she took great delight in informing me that she had become pregnant.

Flower essence for patience: Impatiens (Bach group)

Classic Impatiens people are driven by a constant sense of urgency with an insatiable desire for results. When these results don't come fast enough, such people can become more and more tense and impatient, and less and less tolerant. On the other hand, 'in their positive state,

Impatiens people have much to offer the world in the way of vision, inspiration and the ability to be self-motivated in the pursuit of goals' (Wells, *Essential Flower Essence Book* p. 214).

Negative state
Tense, irritable, with a sense of urgency
Impatiently goal orientated

Positive state
Relaxed; stopping to 'smell the roses'
Patient; process orientated

NB: While Impatiens flower essence helped with the conception process for Kate, this doesn't mean that the remedy is appropriate for all women who are having difficulty becoming pregnant. Although it has been useful for some others in my experience, especially those who are caught up in a fast pace of life, there are many other essences that may assist women who are finding it difficult to conceive, based on their individual personalities and situations.

Male health
Prostate issues

Metaphysically, just as the uterus represents the feminine principle, the prostate represents the masculine principle. This gland secretes a thin, milky, alkaline fluid which acts as a medium to help the sperm on its way to the ovum, for which it competes with other sperm cells. A male who encounters problems associated with the prostate might ask: What do I need to consider about the way I assert or 'package' and present myself? What is my sense of self-worth—what value do I place on myself at this stage in my life? How relevant do I feel? If suffering from an indurated or enlarged prostrate: Have I become too set in the ways I present myself? It's never too late to reinvent or re-create aspects of our Self. For many men, prostrate issues emerge after the age of 50 and in retirement. For some, adapting to a new lifestyle—with its changes in roles and relationships, social life, aims and ambitions—can take them out of their comfort zone and erode self-confidence. In these circumstances, Kangaroo Paw flower essence can help.

Flower essence for adaptability: Kangaroo Paw (Aus Bush group)

Kangaroo paw plants 'display the ability to quickly adapt after bushfires and fill a niche in the environment' (Wells, *Essential Flower Essence Book* p. 220). This capacity is reflected in a positive aspect of Kangaroo Paw flower essence, which fosters the ability to adapt comfortably and confidently on an intimate level to one's environment and people in it.

Negative state
Uncomfortable, awkward and socially 'green'
'Socially insensitive' (Ian White)

Positive state
'Cool' and 'comfortable in your own skin'
Socially adaptable and empathetic

Sexual dysfunction

Another challenge a man may face is sexual impotence. If so, he might ask: How 'potent' do I feel in my work, in my relationships, in my family and life in general? Are there areas where I feel powerless? Self-esteem is an integral part of potency and confidence. Some men try to compensate for underlying low self-esteem through bravado or by acquiring material trappings or status, and in this instance, Sunflower essence (discussed earlier) is useful. On the other hand, others may feel that they don't get enough approval and appreciation or proper recognition and Buttercup flower essence is more appropriate.

Flower essence for a sense of Self-worth: Buttercup (FES group)

Kaminski and Katz (FES) tell us that 'Buttercup can help us appreciate and value ourselves and be unconcerned about kudos or fame.' Buttercup flower essence 'helps us appreciate ourselves and our unique, personal gift to the world' (Wells, *Essential Flower Essence Book* pp. 118–19).

Negative state
Doubting or de-valuing your worth in the world
Unable to recognise and appreciate your unique contribution

Positive state
'Radiant inner light, unattached to outer recognition or fame' (FES)
Sense of place in the greater scheme of things
(Wells, *Essential Flower Essence Book* p. 118)

Digestive system

The state of our physical organs of digestion can provide insights into how we are digesting and assimilating (or not assimilating) our everyday life experiences. When I have a client who is suffering from digestive problems I always ask the obvious: Are you aware of any foods that seem to upset your gut? But then I ask if they aware of any situations, any stresses or any moods that leave them with an upset gut. I help them to answer by asking a hypothetical question: If you were eating out with people you felt uncomfortable being around, would you be more likely to suffer digestive problems than if you were eating the same meal in your comfort zone, perhaps at home with family or friends around whom you felt very comfortable? Invariably the answer is that they would be more likely to have digestive issues after eating with people they don't feel comfortable with. In any situation in which we are not emotionally comfortable we are more inclined to develop physical digestive problems, especially when we are already vulnerable in this area.

On a physical level, the purpose of the digestive system is to recognise nourishing foodstuffs and convert them into simple elements that can be easily absorbed and assimilated into the blood and utilised by various tissues. The gut also filters out and excretes substances that aren't nourishing, along with waste products. On a metaphysical level, the digestive process reflects our ability to filter life experiences and convert them into recognisable elements that can easily be absorbed, assimilated and utilised according to our personal needs and life purposes. We can most easily assimilate what we need from experiences and eliminate or 'let go' of what we don't need when we are inwardly calm and at peace with Self. In this state we are attuned to our 'gut' feelings, intuitively responding to them in a state of FLOW—effortlessly and purposefully immersed in life.

The segments of our digestive tract can inform us about how we are digesting or have digested life experiences, from anticipated experiences in the immediate future, to those being experienced right now, to those that have been experienced recently, to those experienced in the far past. The further we travel down through the digestive tract the more its state/condition can give insight into what we may have *left behind* (or been unable to leave behind) in life. What are we still bothered (or even haunted) by? What past emotional experiences still 'smoulder' and retain 'heat'? What feelings still 'simmer on low' in our psyche? What feelings remain, that we just can't or won't fully let go of? As we will see, the stomach is symbolic of how we greet current and upcoming experiences; the small intestine is symbolic of how we process present, recent and ongoing experiences, how we assimilate the nourishing/positive aspects and accept and release toxic/negative aspects of our experiences; and finally, the colon is symbolic of how well we have discharged, let go, resolved and released the waste products or 'fallout' of our life experiences. Let's take a journey through the gut to explore these ideas in more detail.

The mouth

The condition of our mouth gives insight into how effectively we are responding to our environment—especially verbally. Do we speak up or stay silent when we feel strong emotion? When we have temporarily lost our sense of taste, we might ask: Have I lost my 'taste' for life and what it holds for me now and in the near future? Are there things in my life that have become tasteless? Do I need to consider introducing tasty or tasteful things, or removing tasteless things from my life? OR when we develop a sore tongue and/or red/inflamed areas such as mouth ulcers etc. we might ask: Am I able to articulate exactly what I want from those around me? Do I say what I mean, or do I leave things unsaid? Do I feel free to say what I feel, or do I 'bite my tongue'?

Case study: Mouth ulcers

At one time I used to teach weekend-long seminars, after which I would often develop mouth ulcers within 24 hours of finishing. I wanted to understand why. Sure, taking some Vitamin B complex often helped to clear up the ulcers, but I was much more interested in what caused them to develop in the first place. After research and some soul-searching, I came to the following conclusion. Among the usual 20 or more participants in each seminar there would invariably be one who gradually started to annoy me as the weekend progressed (not their fault—the problem lay in my inability to respond in the moment). At first I would feel only minor irritation but by late on the last day, when I was beginning to tire, I would start to find their questions and antics really annoying. As a professional I had to remain calm and collected on the outside, even though underneath I might be feeling more and more irritated. *I felt powerless or fearful (or some combination of emotions) about saying what I really felt. I literally had to hold (or bite) my tongue!* I worked out that the number and severity of mouth ulcers was directly proportional to how cranky I had become by the end of the weekend, underneath that cool, calm exterior! It was as if, as the weekend progressed, the *unsaid* (and *undead!*) began to eat away at me and my tongue! Incorporating meditation, a few appropriate flower essences, and taking a decent break far from the seminar room at lunchtime proved to be very helpful.

Many of my clients (and some friends) have told me similar stories, often relating to work colleagues who annoyed them. For example, if someone they had to work with was 'bugging' them or 'getting under their skin' and they felt they couldn't honestly address it or speak out about it to those involved, they would eventually pay for it with some negative physical reaction. As my TCM friend would say, 'the body starts to express what a person cannot.'

The stomach

The condition of the stomach gives us insight into how we are greeting upcoming experiences and accepting those being experienced right now. If you often have an upset stomach, you might like to ask: How am I greeting the next moment in my life? Do I have anticipatory anxiety/fear—'butterflies in my stomach'? Am I constantly worried about what is coming up next? Do I dread what life might 'dish up'? Do I lack confidence in my ability to navigate whatever happens? Or am I relaxed and at ease with what I am experiencing right this moment? Am I approaching and navigating what I am experiencing in this or the next moment with acceptance and poise? Do I take a 'que sera sera' approach to life? The answers to these questions will give insight into why we may be developing problems such as discomfort and bloating, acid reflux and dyspepsia, inflammation and ulceration, gut flora imbalance (dysbiosis) etc.

Flower essence for anticipatory anxiety: Garlic (FES group)

Garlic flower essence can be used to help calm the fears that overcome us when we feel that 'the world is our stage' and we are called upon to perform. It helps calm niggling uneasiness as we go about our everyday activities, easing 'butterflies' in the stomach that are associated with anticipatory anxiety (Wells, *Essential Flower Essence Book* p. 186).

Negative state
Over-susceptible to negative environments
Debilitating sense of foreboding

Positive state
Composed, good humoured and 'tuned in'
Dynamic resistance, natural immunity

When we regularly practise meditation, we experience *calm, natural ease and stillness* and become comfortable in the moment—fears and anxieties dissipate. We become more *accepting* of what lies ahead.

The small intestine

The condition of the small intestine gives us insight into how we are processing present, recent and ongoing life experience, i.e. how we are discerning the difference between life experiences that are nourishing/ positive and those that are toxic/negative, so that we can assimilate what is nourishing and release what is toxic. If you are experiencing intestinal bloating and discomfort, pain and/or cramping, IBS, intestinal enzyme disfunction, fermentation and gut flora imbalance, slow bowel transit time (constipation), too rapid transit time (loose stools), ulceration etc, you might ask yourself: Am I ill-at-ease with what I am experiencing? Am I preoccupied, 'churning things over,' *ruminating* and not fully in the present? Am I overwhelmed by what's going on? Am I finding it difficult to 'digest' everything that is happening in and around me? Do I find it difficult to take everything into account and arrive at a decision that FEELS right?

Flower essence for a calm response to life: Dill (FES group)

Dill's aromatic seeds have been used for centuries to treat a wide variety of digestive ailments. (The original baby's colic remedy, called 'gripe water,' contained dill oil.) In its more subtle form as a flower essence, this healing ability helps us better 'digest' and process life experience, assimilating what we need from the environment and discarding what we don't. Rather than be overwhelmed by what is going on around us, it helps restore balance, so we take in only what we need internally, and consume rather than be consumed by what's happening externally!

Negative state
'Overwhelmed due to over-stimulation' (FES)
Hyper-reactive to ('consumed' by) what's around

Positive state
Mutually beneficial environmental exchange
Calmly 'digesting' life, purposeful
(Wells, *Essential Flower Essence Book* p. 167)

Dill can have the effect of allowing you to answer YES to the questions: Am I relaxed and at ease with what I have experienced and am experiencing in life? Am I accepting of what I have experienced and am experiencing, displaying mental clarity and decisiveness when necessary? Practising meditation regularly also helps us to calmly accept all of life's experiences, allowing us to display discernment, and assimilate what we need and let go of what we don't need and/or what doesn't serve us.

Colon/bowel

Simmering in the shadow
Don't let sleeping dogs lie.
You cannot forget what you haven't first remembered;
Heal with an awakened mind's eye.
Then you can say,
'So long, toxic colon.' (Mark Wells)

The condition of the colon gives us insight into how well we have discharged the psychological 'waste-products' of our life experiences. If the processing is not complete, resentment on a conscious or subconscious level can arise from unexpressed and unacted upon emotion when personal needs were unmet. Unresolved ('undigested') issues from the past can ferment and 'eat away' at the depths (or 'bowels') of our being. (One is reminded here of the Jungian concept of the shadow or the underworld realm of Hades in Greek mythology.) 'Deliberate amnesia or mere distance in time and place may mean that the language of events is lost but their emotions roil on in silence and are felt as cravings, aversions, anxieties' (Rockel, 2019 p. 54). If deep feelings remain unresolved we may develop IBS, constipation, diverticulitis, ulcerative colitis, Crohn's disease, malignancies, etc.

Flower essence for freedom from resentment: Willow (Bach group)

Willow grows best beside rivers, creeks and in close proximity to water. The qualities of the water element, which represents emotion, are strongly associated with the willow tree. Unexpressed, suppressed and internalised emotion creates *resentment*, the key word for Willow flower essence. Water is also cleansing and Willow essence helps cleanse our system of emotions that have become stagnant and toxic. Willow helps us to *assimilate* painful experiences, preventing us from becoming stuck in the past, wallowing in pain, sadness or grief. We learn to understand ourselves more deeply and use the wisdom gained to facilitate change in our lives. This is truly 'moving on,' which is very different from denial of past pain. Willow helps us to learn resilience, so that we can delve into our history and use the insights we gain to create a better and more joyous future without feeling victimised by the past (Wells, *Essential Flower Essence Book* p. 370).

Negative state
Victim mentality ('poor me')
Wallowing in resentment

Positive state
Self-determination
Emotional resilience

Willow can help us to *let go* of past trauma by *letting go* of the sense of being wronged and of the indignation felt, bringing deep resilience and the ability to move swiftly towards *acceptance* of what has happened and, therefore, what might happen. It becomes a virtuous cycle. Without acceptance it becomes the opposite, a vicious cycle. Regular practice of meditation also helps us to stay fully conscious of our emotions, even negative ones from the past, long enough to establish a different relationship with them. While in a state of *inner calm, ease and stillness*, we can detach from and observe emotion as something separate from us. We reach such a level of acceptance of the emotion that it loses the negative impact it once had. We understand and take what we need from any emotion we feel and are much wiser for the experience.

The liver

Oh my liver
When rationality checkmates desire,
The edit triggers an internal fire.
A raging hot liver will derange,
But for a state of *flow*
With heart and head united so
To bring the cool change. (Mark Wells)

The liver is the second largest organ in the body, after the skin, and is the second most complex organ after the brain. It performs many crucial functions associated with digestion, immunity, metabolism, and the storage of nutrients. Everything we drink or eat, including medicine, passes through the liver, and when you consider what humans ingest it has a lot to manage and process! No wonder most people's livers are under strain.

We cannot live without our liver.
And living is uncomfortable if our liver doesn't deliver!

Metaphysically, the liver is responsible for managing and processing the *emotional aspect* of life experiences. I often say to clients in consultation: 'Your brain is understanding what I am saying to you at this moment (hopefully!) while your liver is reacting emotionally to what you make of or get from what I am saying.' At a dynamic level, the brain integrates the cognitive understanding aspect, while the liver integrates the feeling response aspect. The brain may or may not recall exactly what happened to you but your liver will never forget how it *felt*!

Unlike other organs, the liver can actually regenerate itself—it has a unique capacity for re-growth after damage. Fortunately, on a metaphysical level the liver can also heal itself when it reviews, processes and releases pain resulting from past trauma, once we learn to let go and face our experiences less reactively: 'My agency, the tiny part of living that belongs to me alone, resides almost entirely in becoming *less reactive and more curious*. And my exercise of this capacity can also alter what I pass on' (Rockel, 2019, p. 54). The ability to become *less reactive and more curious* is especially facilitated by meditation.

We need to *fully* remember and engage with how an experience *felt* before we can fully forget it! It is only then that we can begin to fully let go of the emotional 'heat' associated with painful past experience. To 'let sleeping dogs lie' is to lie to oneself and it does not work, ultimately causing harm to you and others. A word of caution though—*feeling fully* any past trauma can only happen when we are comfortable and strong enough within, and have the appropriate support around us.

The gall bladder

My gall bladder

Do you have the gall to speak it?
Or is the thought untimely,
Or too heated?

To balance and juggle
Tactful and terse
Is the internal struggle
You have come to know.

Be patient.
Reframe it,
But never restrain it.
In time you will find less ebb,
And more *flow*. (Mark Wells)

In Traditional Chinese Medicine, the liver/gall bladder system is intrinsically associated with frustration, anger, and other fiery (yang) emotions, but also with calm, decisive and progressive action—being in the *flow*. If we are frustrated in our attempts to achieve what we desire—what we strongly feel we want in life—we can easily become frustrated, angry, irritable or 'fly off the handle.' Eventually, if we remain stagnant, never engaging with these areas of frustration, at some level we become resentful and *bitter* about our unfulfilled desires and creativity. Our physical liver suffers as a consequence. People who drink heavily, for instance, are invariably suppressing deep frustration. I have often wondered what does more damage to the liver—is it the constant and excessive alcohol passing through, ever over-burdening its detoxification capacity, or is it the suppression of deep emotion, ever over-burdening its (dynamic) emotional processing ability? I believe both these things cause significant harm to the liver! It is interesting to note that bitter-tasting herbs have traditionally been prescribed to help and improve the function of the liver/gall bladder. These herbs usually improve the quality of bile—a very *bitter* secretion—and encourage its proper release from the gall bladder into the digestive tract. To feel *bile* is to feel anger or bitterness toward someone or something. Some traditional sayings relating to the liver provide further insight:

You have an '*angry liver*'—you are very angry.
He was '*livid*'—he was furious.
You are '*a bit liverish*'—you are a bit peeved.
She's '*full of bile*'—she's full of resentment and anger.
I have a '*hot liver*'—I'm irritated and will 'fly off the handle' easily.

And finally, '*I have S.O.L.*' is how one of my clients, a very gentle and refined elderly lady eloquently expressed it. When I described what I thought her digestive and emotional pain might be, she said very softly and deliberately: 'Oh you mean S.O.L.—Shit on the liver.' Lotus flower essence was very helpful for her.

Flower essence for integrated emotionality: Lotus (FES group)

To be effective, spiritual insights need to be grounded in the practicalities of everyday life. Those who benefit from taking Lotus flower essence can sometimes 'think right' but not quite feel right, often because of difficulty in acknowledging that they might be capable of a 'crude and uncivilised' emotion such as anger. Lotus flower essence helps us express the most basic emotions in a practical and creative way. It can help us strike the right balance between the influence of the more 'refined' upper energy centres and the 'cruder' lower ones.

Negative state
'Talking the walk,' head in the clouds
'Spiritual pride'(FES)—inflated and insular sense of self

Positive state
'Walking the talk,' feet on the ground
In touch with our basic feeling nature
Open-minded and inclusive
(Wells, *Essential Flower Essence Book* pp. 231–32)

In summary, if we begin to experience FLOW in our lives, we are able to take decisive action, and frustration, anger and resentment dissipates. A more 'contented liver' can then properly cleanse and enliven the blood flowing through our body.

Circulation

Low blood pressure

Low blood pressure must be taken seriously as it can accompany serious disease conditions that are potentially life threatening. But much of the time, low blood pressure has other causes that aren't due to any underlying disease. For example, it may be part of a family history of benign low blood pressure, or be due to side effects of medication, or even one's individual constitution. Rudolf Steiner said of children who constantly have cold hands (sometimes associated with low blood pressure) that they are taking more time to incarnate and become fully embodied, because of their sensitivity. I am a highly sensitive person (HSP) and I can't remember ever not having cold hands!

If our blood pressure drops too low, the body's vital organs do not get enough oxygen and nutrients, and we can go into shock. This can become life-threatening if not treated. When an individual is approaching death, the systolic blood pressure will typically drop below 95 mm.This is the point of withdrawal from life itself, and from an esoteric standpoint there is no longer a 'will to live.' But low blood pressure alone does not mean that death is imminent. If someone has a history of non-life-threatening low blood pressure, especially when it is accompanied by *vagueness* and disembodied states it would be of value to ask: Does this reflect a lack of personal will, drive or motivation? Has my drive been suppressed for whatever reason, and do I really want to be in the place I find myself in life? Do I need to explore more deeply what I really feel passionate about and what gets my blood flowing? What would enhance my enthusiasm for life, my desire to be involved, and/or what is preventing me from feeling enthusiasm? What would it take to feel deeply and fully committed to a life purpose?

High blood pressure

There are many things that can contribute to the development of high blood pressure, whether temporarily or more permanently. As we age, physiological changes such as loss of elasticity and/or narrowing of blood vessels can impact on and increase blood pressure. Aspects of mind and emotionality can also influence blood pressure positively or negatively. Questions one could ask in relation to high blood pressure are: Am I overreacting to my environment and the persons and/or situations within it? Am I finding that there is too much to do and not enough time to do it in—am I feeling too time-urgent? Am I running out of time in my life to do what I want? Am I letting myself become over-stressed by what is happening around me—even the little things? Do I let things 'get under my skin' too easily? Do I get 'over-heated' and pissed off too easily? Do I often feel a sense of urgency that makes me rush? Do I find it really hard to just stop, let go and relax? Do I, deep down, have a fear of stopping, and standing still for a moment?

- *Systolic pressure* is a measure of the contraction force required by the heart to pump blood around the body. If you have high systolic pressure, you might ask yourself: Am I trying too hard (over-striving)? Do I feel I am always 'pushing shit uphill' and never getting where I want without a struggle?

- High *diastolic pressure* means that the heart is not fully relaxing between beats. One might ask: At a deep level, am I finding it difficult to completely let go? Do I trust in the process of life enough to just let things be, or be more philosophical? Am I trying too hard to control and protect myself against the worst that may happen? No insurance policy can cover everything!!

The skin

The skin is the physiological and metaphysical boundary between what is within and what is outside us. Any physical problem or 'expression' at the skin level can be symbolic of a reaction (physically, emotionally and mentally) to what is happening around us, especially in the immediate and 'felt' environment. A simple example may be when we blush—the skin goes red as a response to something in our immediate environment that has caused us to feel embarrassed or uncomfortable.

In addition, when people are under stress, depressed or enduring other psychological problems, their reaction to their environment will be intensified. In these people their emotional state can exacerbate any already established skin problem or one to which they may be predisposed. Therefore, an environmental trigger, an emotional trigger or both, can 'set off' or aggravate a skin condition. Dr Rick Fried, a psychologist turned dermatologist who is the clinical director of Yardley Dermatology and Clinical Research Associates in Pennsylvania states: 'The common dermatological issues that have been documented to be made worse by stress include acne, rosacea, psoriasis, itching, eczema, pain and hives, just to name a few' (qtd. in Clay, 2015). There is now a field of dermatology called psychodermatology.

I encourage clients to stay positive and hopeful in relation to their skin conditions, which can be unsightly, especially in the eyes of the sufferer, and uncomfortable. I remind them that, although skin symptoms can be part of the pathology of serious ailments, in most cases, symptoms at the skin level are a sign that a health problem is superficial—despite what it looks like! In Traditional Chinese Medicine, health problems confined to the skin are often viewed as a positive sign overall, that the body is resolving potentially more serious health issues, preventing disease affecting internal organs which are more vital for health. According to Hering's Law of Cure, which we will discuss in more detail later, skin symptoms can be regarded as a sign that the disease process is in its final stages when, for example, a rash appears directly after a stressful period in one's life, or the at the end of an illness such as measles (although use of steroid cream may modify the symptom picture and also the outcome). In these two instances the rash satisfies Hering's Law of Cure in three crucial aspects: it appears from the head downwards, moves from within outwards, and moves from major organs to minor organs. Of course, all health conditions should be closely monitored by a health professional with medical training.

As mentioned, for a significant number of my clients, skin 'break outs' have signalled that the stress they have been experiencing is now on the decline (similar to migraine sufferers who tend to experience migraines more often at the end of an intensely stressful period). Having weathered the storm a client can now address the repercussions.

Flower essence for calm during intensity: Indian Pink (FES group)

I have found that Indian Pink flower essence has—*not* coincidentally—often been indicated when a client was experiencing an emotionally inflammatory reaction to their life situation that has also manifested in the skin. When we feel that outside influences have encroached on our *personal space* to the point where we are *torn in many directions*, losing our orientation and focus, we should consider Indian Pink flower essence. The flower's rich, blood-red colour is significant. It signals the flower essence's ability to address *acute, inflammatory, red-raw and 'angry'* reactions in the mind and body to stressors in the immediate environment.

Negative state
Psychically 'frayed at the edges'; *inflamed*
'Inability to stay centred during intense activity' (FES)

Positive state
'Managing and coordinating diverse forms of activity' (FES)
Calm focus in the midst of heightened activity
(Wells, *Essential Flower Essence Book* pp. 217–18)

When clients have heightened or inflamed mental/emotional responses to the environment and this manifests on the physical level in the form of *acute* inflammatory reactions, especially of the skin, I have often found that Scarlet Monkeyflower essence is indicated along with Indian Pink. With Scarlet Monkeyflower there is decidedly more fear and discomfort associated with the emotion of anger, and a greater incentive to avoid it in oneself and others than with Indian Pink. Indian Pink is more commonly prescribed for temporary and transient conditions of the mind, whereas Scarlet Monkeyflower helps those with conditions that affect the mind more deeply. In my experience, Indian Pink is for more acute/short-lived conditions and Scarlet Monkeyflower is for more chronic/constitutional conditions.

Meditation and reactive emotions

Regular meditation helps you change your relationship with all your emotions, especially intense and reactive responses to your immediate environment. Increasing awareness of one's *calm, natural ease and stillness within* subdues intense emotional reactions. In this way, it helps you manage stresses much better and therefore helps those whose skin conditions are influenced and made worse by stress. Your deep, emotional reactions to what is happening around you remain a great source of information to you, without the previous negative impact on health. You become wiser about what it is in your environment that is really 'getting to you' and what to do about it!

Immune system

One thing I have always found interesting in my academic studies over four decades is the way the subject of Immunology has consistently and significantly changed over the years—from my first lessons in Immunology as part of my Biological Sciences degree, to my studies a decade later for an Applied Science degree in Naturopathy, to studies another decade on for my Master of Social Sciences. You could say, 'Gee, isn't that great, the pace at which the science of Immunology is evolving!' But at the same time, these changes have confirmed for me our short-lived security of knowledge regarding any definitive understanding of Immunology. As a result, I don't have a huge amount of confidence in the current scientific understanding of how our natural immune system functions, what enhances it and what undermines it. I have always been a restless seeker after understanding about natural principles and truths that have integrity and, most importantly, that have stood the test of time—things that applied thousands of years ago and will apply thousands of years into the future. As a result, I was naturally drawn to Nature Cure philosophy and practice. (And in fact, the Nature Cure will be the subject of my next book!!)

As a practising naturopath who finds ways to apply the Nature Cure every day, I have always found that the best way to help my clients' natural immune system to function at its optimum is to take a broad view, which encompasses physical, emotional and psychological aspects of their wellbeing. In this way I can help to protect them against potential threats on all these levels. Rather than identify specific threats such as susceptibility to a particular virus or type of emotional stress, I firstly look at whether the state of a client's *general susceptibility* to their environment is *normal or abnormal*. This approach is underpinned by one of naturopathy's fundamental principles regarding disease: '*It's the soil not the germ*.' If the 'soil'—the person's overall health and wellbeing—is of good quality, then the 'germ'—the virus, the emotional stress etc.—will have minimal impact and the person's natural and innate self-recuperative powers will manage and successfully navigate it.

A pathogen's virulence or potential to do damage, like the potential negative impact of psychological stress, is directly related to our state of overall health and wellbeing, i.e. our unique *susceptibility*. From the point of view of a national health system, assessing the health of each individual in a population is almost impossible, and that is why we necessarily make 'one size fits all' decisions when it comes to disease protection measures such as vaccination. There are, however, opportunities for people to be proactive about seeking qualified health practitioners who are skilled at holistic assessment. From this perspective, a person's idiosyncratic symptoms and qualities reflect their current level of susceptibility—that is, their inherent vulnerability to disease-inducing factors such as bacteria, viruses, stress and environmental toxins, and their potential ability to heal and protect themselves.

Normal susceptibility which is reflected in natural good health and emotional wellbeing, keeps us protected from disease. *Abnormal or altered susceptibility* (see below)—due to less-than-optimal health and less-than-optimal emotional wellbeing—makes us more vulnerable and quicker to succumb to 'germs' such as viruses, stresses etc.

Signs of abnormal or altered susceptibility

- Absence of occasional acute, rapid-onset, short-lasting illnesses (e.g. a head cold) followed by complete recovery.
- Chronic disease is present.
- The individual is permanently medicated for chronic illness, or regularly takes other medication in some form.
- Addiction is present.
- Poor diet (e.g. excess processed food) is a feature.
- Poor lifestyle (inadequate movement/exercise, rest, play, sleep).
- High sensitivity that is badly managed.
- The individual experiences ongoing high stress levels and/or has had significant past emotional trauma.
- There is a lack of flow, and little sense of purpose/meaning and/or creative expression; there are feelings of discontent.
- Active, inherited, constitutional weaknesses and vulnerabilities are present.
- There is regular exposure to extreme environmental conditions (cold, heat etc.).

To enhance natural immunity, the whole person—their physical, emotional and mental health and their diet and lifestyle—must be assessed and brought as much as possible into alignment with the natural laws of healthy living. From this book's perspective, *emotional* healing and wellbeing is as important, if not more important than anything else when it comes to healthy natural living.

Cancer/malignancy

I should precede this discussion by saying that as a practising naturopath and counsellor I don't treat cancer in any direct way. I treat the *whole person*. And when I take this approach, anything is possible, especially better overall health outcomes. Of course, the signs and symptoms of current illness are very much taken into account within an overall and in-depth assessment carried out in a consultation. Any health practitioner needs to understand each client's current pathology and its associated prognosis. Also, every client I have treated who had cancer, has also necessarily been under the care and guidance of an appropriate medical physician.

Dr Ainslea Meares, a Melbourne psychiatrist who practised throughout the second half of the 20th century, taught his own form of meditation to many clients who had been diagnosed with cancer, guiding them individually and in groups at his clinic. As a psychiatrist and physician, he conducted a full physical examination as well as an in-depth psychological assessment of each patient and therefore developed a deep understanding of their situation. Dr Meares's perspective on cancer, gained primarily from his work with patients and his own investigations and research, rings true with my experience as a practitioner. He found that significant psychological and emotional factors are implicit in the disease state for those diagnosed with cancer.

> The first layer we encounter in the unconscious is what Jung called the shadow ... parts of ourselves we don't like, *don't know, or don't want to know*. The shadow can be repressed in us like a cancer ...[but] the positive can show us a meaningful part of ourselves we should recognise and *live out*. (Dunne, 2015 p. 106)

Dr Meares's patients practised meditation not as an alternative to conventional treatment but mostly in conjunction with it. Regular meditation took a few patients through to cure, and others experienced remission from cancer. For most, though, it brought a significant improvement in quality of life irrespective of the final outcome. Research by Mehta et al. (2019) found that mindfulness meditation is being used increasingly in many aspects of cancer management, where its usefulness has been confirmed by multiple trials. Continuing research shows that the main evidence of benefit of mindfulness meditation in cancer is to reduce toxicity (especially associated with cancer treatments) and stress. This is consistent with the views of Dr Meares who witnessed at his clinic how intensive meditation had a positive influence on all aspects of health and wellbeing of those suffering from cancer. His approach to meditation has been carried forward into the 21st century, and is still taught by Pauline McKinnon, an acknowledged expert who remains true to his original method, which she now refers to as Stillness Meditation Therapy (SMT). Her website—stillnessmeditation. com.au—provides a wealth of information.

This strong anecdotal evidence and the growing body of scientific evidence in the area of mindfulness and meditation for cancer patients is very encouraging. A summary of Meares's findings gained from many years of work with cancer diagnosed patients is as follows:

- Many patients had experienced an 'out of the usual,' intense stress in the two years prior to their diagnosis.

- The patients felt that they couldn't say or do anything about their stress—'don't know or don't want to know.' They felt powerless and couldn't 'live it out.'

- Stress was not the sole cause of patients' disease but when acting with other factors, e.g. smoking, diet and lifestyle, it provided a very significant trigger in bringing on the development of cancer.

Dr Meares often used his poetry to convey insights gained through working with cancer diagnosed patients:

On how the cancer started

Think back
Think back a little,
Six to eighteen months
Before the first signs of it.
Many recall
A period of increased tension.
Some real problem
Causing great worry and distress.
Some stress,
Far more than average,
With resulting anxiety and depression.
Of being caught in a situation
From which there is no escape.
Of course we all have our troubles,
But this story comes so consistently
That it strongly suggests
A psychological factor
In the cause of cancer. (Ainslea Meares)

From my experience with clients, I would make one addition to Meares's conclusions and broaden the scope of predisposing factors to include emotional trauma from as far back as childhood. For those affected, the sense of *powerlessness* has been internalised, modified and disguised as secondary maladaptive responses and behaviours.

Anxiety makes our body react
With more [cortisol]
To cope with the stress
Which is all to the good
But the extra [cortisol]
Upsets our immune response
And abnormal cells,
Which would have been killed,
Are now allowed to grow. (Ainslea Meares)

Hering's Law of Cure

I would like to refer once more to Hering's Law of Cure, a significant principle in naturopathic/Nature Cure philosophy. Dr Constantine Hering (1800–1880) was a medical doctor and homeopath who formulated a four-point guide to the dynamics of recovery and the *right direction of cure*. Hering's Law allowed physicians and homeopaths to track their patients' recovery and judge whether they were progressing *towards* or *away from* cure, towards chronic disease. Though the use of contemporary pharmaceutical drugs has modified how disease symptoms are expressed, and this can make it more difficult to perceive the direction of cure, Hering's Law is still informative about the actual disease trajectory.

1 We heal from the head down

Before we can begin to heal we must have faith in our ability to heal. Deep healing must start at the mental and emotional level and this prepares us for physical healing. The message in the body—the intrinsic in the extrinsic—gives us clues about where to start.

2 We heal from within outwards

Symptoms move from the interior of the body outwards to the exterior, to the skin and extremities.

3 We heal from the most vital organs to the least vital organs

Symptoms move from the more vital organs (e.g. lungs or liver) to the less vital organs (e.g. skin or mucous membranes)

4 We heal in reverse order as the symptoms have appeared or been suppressed

This means that the last problem someone has (or presents with) is the first problem to improve/disappear, and then previous problems, in reverse order of their appearance, are resolved and healed.

Suppression—a summary

Emotions inform and motivate action, prompting us to respond in the short term, and adapt, grow, and develop in the long term. However, when emotions are suppressed by being stifled, unacted upon and left unresolved, they can start to impact negatively on our emotional and physical wellbeing. As an example, if you intimidate a child into not crying just in the moment they are about to cry after becoming upset about something, you have suppressed the child's active, physical response to a *primary* emotion felt as a result of that negative experience. The basic emotional needs that made them want to cry are not given a full opportunity to be expressed and find some closure. The impact on the child going forward is entirely in proportion to the degree of emotional hurt felt at the time. If the child is sensitively supported and their emotional needs are met, they are likely to be easily distracted from crying over a minor issue, and the emotional impact is likely to be also minor and insignificant. However, if a child's crying response is immediately suppressed when they have experienced a significant emotional hurt, this suppression of a primary emotional response can give rise to complex maladaptive emotions and dysfunctional behaviours.

This is analogous to when physical symptoms of disease are suppressed without acknowledging and attending to their root cause(s). Just as the child's crying is an action in response to a primary emotional hurt felt from deeper within, physical symptoms of disease are generally the body's expression of its response to disease deeper within—*not* the full disease itself, and sometimes they are just the tip of the iceberg. If we ignore the internal sources of disease and just treat (that is, suppress) the external disease symptoms, a potential is created for more serious and/or chronic health problems to develop.

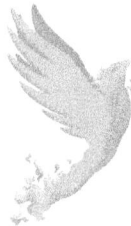

EMOTION–THOUGHT
–ACTION

I n most cases, it is difficult, if not impossible, to consciously identify whether a thought precedes an emotion or vice versa—it is a bit like asking, 'Which came first, the chicken or the egg?' Studies show evidence for both orders of occurrence. I believe it probably comes down to the way each individual uniquely perceives their experiences in the world. My personal experience is that my emotions—especially what I have referred to before as the 'felt sense'—precede my thoughts, but I am a highly sensitive person (HSP)!

The relationship between emotion and thought

My experience with and understanding of felt-sense *interoception* is that our brain, and then our thinking, respond initially to our conscious and unconscious emotional and sensory responses—what is 'felt'—within the many dimensions of our being. To gain further understanding, it will be interesting to follow the results of research that is accumulating in the area of the gut-brain axis—the bidirectional communication between the central nervous system and the enteric nervous system, which links emotional and cognitive centres of the brain with peripheral intestinal functions.

The fact that I have been so drawn to flower essence therapy, emotion-focused therapy, and Jungian psychotherapy tells you of my regard for the primary importance these therapies give to feelings and emotions. Carl Jung believed that what we feel is a huge part of what makes us human. My observation is that society places much emphasis on the cultivation and development of intellect, especially through our educational institutions, but far less on our emotional and spiritual nature. Feelings and emotions are often devalued and/or repressed (although Steiner education attempts to address this imbalance). What we feel, and how we interpret it, has a very profound impact on our life; feelings are as important and as real, if not more real, than our thinking. Awareness and understanding of our unique and distinctive sensations and emotions is a key to what Jung calls individuation—the discovery of our individual Self-identity and capacity for Self-realisation. As we grow personally, we become more aware that what we feel is not quite the same as emotion. While emotion does include feeling, we can feel something without getting emotional about it. This felt sense is often called *intuition*—something we can learn to trust more and more.

There is no doubt that thoughts can provoke emotions, and depression for instance can be maintained and exacerbated by negative thoughts. Thoughts and emotions can 'feed' off each other in a vicious cycle, when a negative emotion gives rise to negative thoughts, and negative thoughts in turn increase negative emotions (Teasdale & Barnard, 1993). Becoming aware of our tendency to get attached to thinking patterns to the point where we cannot separate ourselves from our thoughts—referred to as *fusion*—is a key element in meditative *acceptance* therapies like Acceptance and Commitment Therapy (Hayes, Strosahl, & Wilson, 2004) and mindfulness-based stress reduction (Kabat-Zinn, 1990). In these therapies, clients learn to observe their thoughts (and feelings), and rather than fusing with them and so believing them to be true, clients learn to stand back and witness thoughts as something separate—defusing from them—so that there is more possibility of choice about how to interpret and respond to experiences.

Thoughts and emotions in a vicious cycle

Feeling frustration after something goes wrong
leads to THOUGHTS such as
'I've got to stop feeling this way but ...'
which leads to feeling *less hopeful* ... feeling *more frustrated.*

Defusing from thoughts in a virtuous cycle

Feeling frustration after something goes wrong
leads to THOUGHTS such as
'I will learn from this experience'
and this leads to feeling *more hopeful* ... feeling *less frustrated*.

FET is a very potent tool to help people *defuse from* negative thoughts.

Flower essence for defusing from thoughts: Scotch Broom (FES group)

Scotch Broom flower essence enables us to develop a more positive outlook overall so that we can *defuse from* our negative thoughts during difficult or challenging times.

Negative state
Discouraged and disheartened; hopeless
Pessimism about the world (FES)
[Depressed feelings *fused with* negative thoughts]

Positive state
Seeing difficulties/challenges as opportunities for growth; hopeful
'Positive and optimistic feelings about the world' (FES)
[*Defused from* negative thoughts]
(Wells, *Essential Flower Essence Book* p. 308)

EMOTIONS AND THEIR ACTION TENDENCIES

Emotions create urges that motivate us to action—they inform our *action tendencies*—allowing us to physically respond in the short term, and adapt, grow, and develop in the long term. Anger, for example, can create a determined urge to defend or attack, and fear can create the urge to avoid or escape. As we have seen, these urges can be adaptive or maladaptive depending on the situation. They become problematic/ maladaptive when people follow them without a conscious decision to do so—this is what we refer to as impulsive behaviour.

Impulsive behaviour is the immediate result of an emotion, but most often a person is UNAWARE that this is the case—they are *mindless*—and have no choice about their response. And though there is usually some immediate benefit from satisfying a strong impulsive urge, this satisfaction is short lived and the negative repercussions are experienced soon afterwards. For example, over-indulging in comfort food, though satisfying in the moment, may be followed immediately by a feeling of guilt (or indigestion or both), and later on by a detrimental impact on health and wellbeing. Also, because the urge can only be temporarily satisfied, it doesn't take long to return. A sugar hit usually guarantees another will be required soon, when blood-sugar levels over-compensate and drop even further than before the first sugar intake.

Impulsive actions that result from emotions underlie a wide range of issues, including eating problems, violence and addiction. They are often associated with maladaptive behaviours arising from *secondary reactive emotions* (discussed earlier) that have developed after the *actions* required to meet past primary emotional needs have been left unmet. In response to negative or uncomfortable emotions—on a conscious or unconscious level—a person may *automatically* start to eat, in a process called emotional eating (Konttinen, 2020), which is also an intrinsic aspect of binge eating.

Impulsive behaviours are more likely to occur during stressful times. A person trying to deal with stress-induced emotion may become overwhelmed, unable to think clearly, and may then become aggressive and offend someone with what they say. Another person's *impulsive* response may be to start eating. Impulsive behaviour can be regarded as the opposite to *autonomous*, self-regulated behaviour in which people feel in control of their lives because they consciously make choices and take responsibility for their actions.

Becoming more *aware*—more *mindful*—of the action tendencies that are generated by an emotional state is a powerful way to reduce impulsive action. Using *mindful* attention through meditation practice to become aware of the emotional urges behind action tendencies helps to create space—a *pause* that allows us to maintain composure—between feeling an emotion in response to an experience, and the reaction that follows. Rather than impulsively acting upon emotion, mindful awareness of the action tendencies that accompany the emotion creates space for self-reflection, which disrupts an automatic pattern of responding. This space or pause created for choice can be used to engage in behaviour that is likely to promote health and wellbeing rather than reduce it.

Meditation, flower essences, and impulsivity

Mindfulness is an extremely beneficial by-product of meditation. It enables us to be broad-minded enough to perceive more choices at any given time. Research findings show that mindfulness is less associated with impulsivity (*automatic action* that gives *no choice*), and more associated with conscious, self-regulated action (*autonomous action* that allows for *choice*) (Fetterman et al., 2010).

Appropriately chosen flower essences in FET can help us to stand back, observe and engage in a *mindful pause*, rather than reacting in a 'knee-jerk,' impulsive manner when certain urges/desires emerge. Flower essences enable us to make better decisions and choices about what actions we take, and this results in better, more adaptive outcomes.

Flower essence for mindful response to impulses: Apricot (FES group)

Apricot is a flower essence that enables us to understand and be more *mindful* of the emotional needs that are asking to be satisfied, behind our impulsive actions, especially around sugar consumption.

Negative state
Strong, impulsive cravings, especially for sugar/sweets
Lack of 'sweetness and lightness' in life

Positive state
Mindful, personal insight about cravings
Life is sweetened with emotional nourishment
(Wells, *Essential Flower Essence Book* p. 91)

Many people try to use willpower alone to control their tendencies toward impulsive action, but this is usually ineffective. Research consistently shows that when people exert self-control through will alone, this results in decreased self-control in subsequent tasks. For example, when a dieter says 'no' to a tempting piece of pie, that dieter is more likely to fail in refusing chocolate not so long after. Controlling oneself—in this case controlling the urge to eat—requires cognitive and emotional self-regulatory resources that soon become exhausted and unavailable for later attempts.

This unsustainability of self-regulatory resources was displayed in a study by Alberts et al. (2012) in which a number of participants were asked to watch a distressing video. Three groups were created. One group was asked to apply self-control and suppress all emotions felt during the video. Another group was asked to apply mindful acceptance (mindfulness), to allow emotions to be present, and to acknowledge and observe them. Participants in the last group did not receive any instructions and were just asked to watch the movie. After the movie, all participants completed a computer task that required self-control. It was found that participants who suppressed their emotions performed worst on this second, post-movie self-control task. In contrast, participants who accepted their emotions mindfully while watching the video, outperformed both of the other groups. These findings also provide insight into one of the mechanisms underlying *mindful acceptance*, namely that it probably conserves our emotional self-regulatory resources.

Meditation and self-regulation

As mentioned, one of the many capacities people develop through regular practice of meditation is *mindful acceptance*. This conserves emotional self-regulatory resources through acceptance of the emotions that are present. This then conserves overall energy, and so vitality is sustained and resilience is more assured. Very strict or 'crash' diets that require much self-control/willpower often help people lose weight rapidly, but they almost invariably relapse. Emotional self-regulatory resources quickly become exhausted, and a vicious cycle of dieting and relapse into bingeing on whatever the diet restricted can easily develop.

Flower essence for flexible Self-regulation: Rock Water (Bach group)

Rock Water is particularly suited to those who are *overly* self-disciplined, self-controlled and self-regulated in their behaviour. In my book, *The Bach Flowers Today* (2013), I describe a day in the life of a person who could definitely benefit from taking Rock Water essence:

> A client comes with major concerns about his general health. He describes his daily routine—up at exactly 6.02 a.m., beginning the day with 20 minutes' meditation; at 6.22 a.m. a 15-minute brisk walk; at 6.37 a.m. a bowel movement until complete evacuation takes place (the quality of the whole day being dependent on this process); breakfast is a large bowl of muesli made from exactly weighed amounts of raw ingredients—the recipe coming from the book that also outlines the rest of his daily regime—and so on, until bedtime at precisely 10.02 p.m.

Needless to say this textbook lifestyle takes more out of him than it gives. He, and to a lesser extent everyone around him, has become a victim of his own rigid regimentation, giving up all his freedoms in pursuit of a way of life that has worked beautifully for someone else. Unfortunately, many people with this pattern of rigidity succumb to bingeing behaviour when their emotional self-regulatory resources become exhausted.

Negative state
Obsession with ideals
Rigid formality; extreme self-regulation

Positive state
Flexibility and open-mindedness; mindful acceptance
Adaptability (Wells, *Essential Flower Essence Book* p. 294)

Self-control/willpower alone is usually not enough to achieve lasting change. When people exert extreme and unnatural self-control, this can result in a decrease in self-control in other areas of their life, when their self-regulatory resources fatigue. I believe this applies especially when the emotional urges being suppressed are natural and instinctive, such as those associated with our sexuality. If there is no way of expressing these desires, their suppression requires enormous cognitive self-regulatory resources that eventually become depleted. This provides insight into the ghastly sexual abuse of children perpetrated by some members of the clergy. During my experience of being educated in the Catholic schooling system, I knew of a few clergy who were found guilty of sexually abusing students. My observation of these abusers was that they were extremely self-disciplined and self-regulated—until they weren't! When their self-regulatory resources failed, they engaged in horrendous behaviour. Of course, there are other factors in many instances where clergy have abused those in their care, as when there has been organised and premeditated grooming of vulnerable people.

POSITIVE EMOTIONS: THE BROADENING AND UNDOING EFFECT
The negative downward spiral

Although as discussed earlier, so-called 'negative' emotions can play a vital and adaptive role, relentless experience of these emotions in an intense form can become harmful to health, increasing the risk of heart disease (Fredrickson et al., 2000) and many other health issues. Negative emotions cause a *narrowing* of perspective to focus on the specifics of a problem. Fear, for instance, causes the individual to prepare for fight or flight, an ancestrally adaptive response. This function of negative emotions is undoubtedly adaptive in life-threatening situations that require quick, decisive and very specific action in a narrow window of opportunity. However, this function becomes maladaptive in non-threatening situations because the instinctive action tendency is fixed and therefore *mindless*.

The *narrowing effect* of negative emotions on one's focus can trigger self-perpetuating, vicious cycles of thinking, feeling, and behaving that are maladaptive, eventually reducing health and wellbeing. An example of the downward, narrowing spiral of feeling and thinking is when sadness causes someone to focus excessively on the negative side of an event and this then triggers other negative feelings, such as anger, insecurity, and frustration. In turn, these feelings can lead to social withdrawal that leads to more sad feelings and further rumination, and so the vicious cycle continues. Over time, this negative spiral of thinking, feeling, and behaving can result in pervasive self-limiting beliefs about the world and oneself: 'I am worthless,' 'I have nothing to offer,' 'Others ignore me,' 'I have no control over my life,' and so the negative spiral intensifies.

It is important to note here that a negative spiral is NOT an inevitable consequence of a 'negative' emotion such as fear or anger. Rather, a negative spiral reflects an individual's inability to effectively manage emotion and its impact. Narrowing effects on behaviour and cognition that are triggered by maladaptive emotions such as the 'glass half empty' response, can be counteracted by a 'glass half full' response. New, *positively adaptive emotions* can be introduced to transform a maladaptive emotional state.

Emotion-focused therapy (EFT) posits that emotions themselves have an innately adaptive potential that can change problematic emotional states and interactions. Emotion is an innate adaptive system that has evolved to help people not only survive but also thrive. Primary emotions are connected to our most essential needs, and EFT is an approach designed to help clients become aware and make productive use of their emotions by 'accessing the important information and *meanings* about themselves and their world that emotions provide' (Greenberg, 2017). EFT helps clients discern how to introduce *adaptive/ positive emotions* to transform their maladaptive/negative emotions, and how to self-regulate emotions that overwhelm them. Both meditation and flower essence therapy can help people with this process. Flower essence therapy and meditation assist people to *broaden* their perspective, and this enables their moment-to-moment, more mindful, thought-to-action repertoire to expand. After taking flower essences and/or meditating regularly, clients often say things like, 'I was able to stand back from a situation, observe myself, and act differently than before. And things worked out better!'

The positive upward spiral

According to Fredrickson's Broaden and Build theory (1998), the function of positive emotions differs fundamentally from the function of negative emotions. In contrast to the narrowing effect of negative emotions, positive emotions cause a *broadening* of perspective that expands the thought-to-action repertoire, and allows more choice about ways of responding than a neutral or fearful/anxious state. Positive emotions cause people to experience a wider than usual field of attention that is more *mindful* and includes increased cognition. This greater range of ideas and concepts also leads to stronger action urges towards things one wants to do or is willing to try. Experience of positive emotions prompts individuals to discard automatic, knee-jerk behavioural scripts, making more room for choice and the pursuit of novel and diverse, spontaneous and unscripted paths of thought and action.

Imagine waking up *feeling positive* and excited about the day ahead—you 'get up on the right side of the bed'! On a morning like this, you are more likely than usual to notice a beautiful sky while walking to work (broadened attention), more likely at work to come up with novel ideas in a meeting, more likely to think of ways to assist your clients (broadened cognition), and more likely to have different ideas about what you want to do after finishing work (broadened action urges). In contrast, if you 'get up on the wrong side of the bed,' *feeling resentful* about going to work and lacking motivation, you are more likely to become annoyed if someone bumps into you because they're on their phone, not paying attention and walking on the wrong side of the footpath. You then walk on expecting more of the same (narrowed attention) and as a consequence, miss the shop windows you usually like glancing into and don't notice your favourite public gardens as you pass them. Then you start to think about how careless and inconsiderate people are, and wonder, 'What's the point?' (narrowed cognition). You have no creative ideas about what to do at work or afterwards because of your negative mood (narrowed action urges)!

Emotions can have a direct impact on the way we perceive and relate to the world. While negative emotions tend to narrow our way of responding, positive emotions tend to broaden our responses and interactions with the environment, allowing us to 'open up' and engage in a more dynamic and proactive way.

Broadening effects of positive emotions:

- Positive emotions *broaden the scope & quality of visual attention* so that people detect more nuanced information in their visual field, (Fredrickson & Branigan, 2005). People who look at their lives in a more contextual way maintain a better perspective.
- Positive emotions *increase creativity* (Rowe et al., 2007; Isen 1987) *and expand the repertoire of desired actions (divergent thinking)* to include more problem solving and creative possibilities.
- Positive emotions *expand a person's openness to new experiences (broad-mindedness)* (Kahn & Isen, 1993).
- Positive emotions *increase openness to receiving critical feedback (open-mindedness)* (Raghunathan & Trope, 2002).
- Positive emotions *increase the sense of 'oneness' with close others (inclusiveness)* (Waugh & Fredrickson, 2006). People who regularly practise meditation often report a greater sense of 'oneness' with their environment and all of humanity.
- Positive emotions *'widen peoples' outlook in ways that, little by little, beneficially reshape who they are' (personal growth)* (Frederickson & Kurtz, 2011, p. 36).

Flower essences and the broadening effect:

- Star Tulip *broadens the scope of visual attention.*
- Iris *expands the repertoire of desired actions.*
- Indian Paintbrush *increases creativity.*
- Purple Monkeyflower *expands a person's openness to new experiences.*
- Calendula *increases openness to critical feedback.*
- Quaking Grass *increases the sense of 'oneness' with close others.*
- Sagebrush *widens peoples' outlooks in ways that, little by little, beneficially reshape who they are.*

Positive emotions have immediate but also long-lasting effects on cognition and behaviour. The broadening of the field of attention, thoughts, and action urges helps the individual to explore new ideas and novel actions and this has a flow-on effect on many aspects of life. For example, the experience of positive emotions may cause a person to try out a new activity such as joining a sporting team. Because they have optimism—positive emotions—about the benefits of being part of the club, they are motivated to endure their initial nervousness and discomfort—negative emotions—about not knowing anyone, and their doubts about their sporting prowess. In time, being part of a team allows them to build their health and fitness, and gain emotional and social intelligence skills. They expand their social network, learn resilience by bouncing back after losing a match or recovering from an injury, and improve their physical skills and adaptability. The club and its members become a permanent resource which can be accessed when coping with difficult life situations. When facing stress or setbacks, they draw from abilities gained as part of the team, and can talk things through with a team member who has experienced similar ups and downs. The experience of positive emotions increases confidence in their ability to cope, and a continued cycle of positive emotions assures the development of greater resilience.

Case study: Migraine

I will use my own experience to exemplify how I was able to use the *broadening effect* of positive emotions to bring about profound changes in my life. I used to suffer with very painful migraines from the age of eight through to my mid-twenties. The first phase of a migraine is known as the premonitory phase or 'preheadache'—it signals that a headache is about to start and in my case, it took the form of a visual signal, a flickering, jagged arc of light causing a temporary blind spot. For many years, as soon as this occurred I would panic and start to catastrophise—a learned maladaptive emotional response—because the preheadache signalled imminent pain and incapacitation.

One day, though, I woke up after a migraine had passed, and realised that although I did still have a slightly sore head I generally felt much calmer, more relaxed and less anxious than in the preceding days. I also noted that this had been the pattern in the past, and that I usually experienced this feeling of calm and peace of mind for a number of days after a migraine. I asked myself, What could this mean? Could it be that my migraines were serving a purpose, slowing me down so that I could recompose myself through a kind of rebooting of my nervous system, to start up again from a calmer, less aroused state? I began to make sense of why *my* migraines occurred, and this more positive and curious *reappraisal* changed my attitude toward them significantly. It allowed me to *reframe* them in the context of my overall health and wellbeing, so that a more *broad-minded* and holistic view became possible. I now recognised that my migraines no longer just represented a random period of pain and suffering but also an impending period of calm and reduced anxiety, a sort of light at the end of a tunnel. A new *meaning* for my ailment had been established in my mind. Positive (adaptive) emotions had been added to the mix of my overall experience.

From that point onwards, my catastrophising and bracing against the arrival of the visual cue of an imminent headache started to decrease. I realised that catastrophising increased my nervous tension and anxiety and this increased my pain levels and need for medication. Now, when the visual cues appeared, I still had the expectation of pain, but at the same time I had a positive expectation of feeling much better afterwards. It crossed my mind that if I never had migraines, I would never get respite from the tense and anxious state that I unfortunately had become accustomed to.

It remained true that a big weekend of drinking—this was my early twenties!—or eating chocolate would often trigger a migraine, but now my positive take, backed up by real-life experience, allowed me to develop more and more acceptance and engage less and less in expecting the worst. With this, the pain of the migraines gradually lessened. With less pain, less painkilling medication was required, and so I would also feel more clear-headed the following day. I also began to wonder about the long term health effects of suppressing migraines with medication, if I didn't or couldn't change the state of my nervous system. Would I develop more chronic and deep-seated nervous problems? Would I need more and more medication? These considerations gave me more incentive to become less dependent on painkillers.

I now recognised that things like alcohol and chocolate were only triggers for my migraines and, from a holistic perspective, not underlying causes or predisposing factors. If I was going to eliminate migraines from my life I would need to eliminate their cause(s) and change my predisposition to them. Fortunately, finding new meaning for *my* migraines opened up many possibilities for me. With a more optimistic view came more opportunities to influence not only my experience of migraine but also my nervous tension and anxiety. This led me to focus on how I might naturally achieve a more permanent state of calm, with less tension and anxiety—the very thing that my body/mind was achieving on a regular basis through painful migraines. I started to explore other (far less painful!) ways to alleviate nervous tension and anxiety. This was life-changing because it opened up many natural health avenues to explore, providing possibilities relating to my migraines but also my overall life direction at a time when I really needed to develop a greater sense of purpose. I became more and more inspired as I took these first steps on what became a lifelong journey, which I still follow passionately today, studying and practising different approaches to healing, health and wellbeing.

I learned relaxation techniques and began to meditate regularly. I also began to use natural medicines, and within six months my migraines had become very infrequent and much less intense. Within twelve months they were no longer part of my life! All throughout that year I gained much understanding of myself and grew personally from experiencing all the dimensions of my illness, being able to sense and connect with its deeper *meaning*—the 'message in the body.' '*Positive (adaptive) emotions widen people's outlooks in ways that, little by little, beneficially reshape who they are*' (Frederickson & Kurtz, 2001, p. 36). The following diagram shows how the *broadening effect helped me to change myself* and ultimately be rid of my migraines. Good riddance I say!

Figure 4: The broadening effect—my experience with migraine

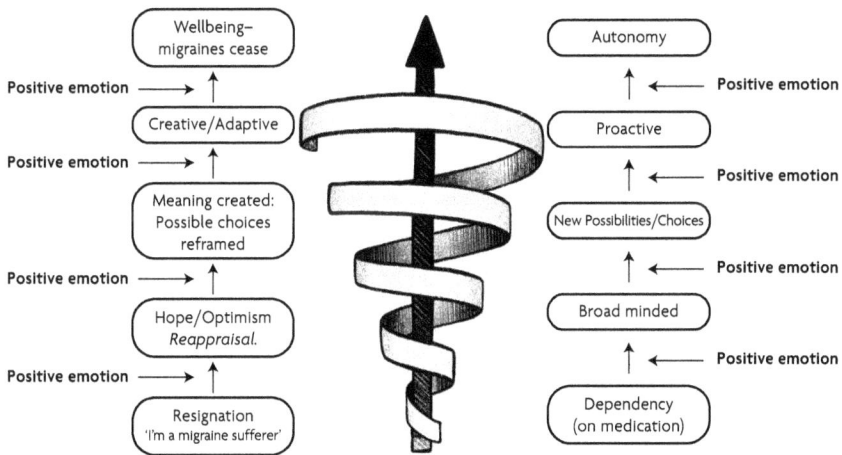

The 'undoing' effect

According to the *build hypothesis*, increasing and maintaining the experience of positive emotions over time allows people to build durable resources that can help them navigate and even *undo* the impact of negative emotional experiences (past and present). Let's look at an example of how experiencing positive emotions directly counteracts (*undoes*) negative impacts—maladaptive effects—of negative emotions. Many of us know how even the thought of public speaking can increase our anxiety levels, resulting in our body and mind going into a state that prepares us for specific actions such as fight or flight, or freeze. Positive emotions have been found to *undo* this unnecessary preparation that is unhealthy and can be incapacitating. It is interesting to note here that a significant number of people regard their fear of public speaking as being greater than their fear of death. I was almost, though not quite, in that category!

In an experiment by Fredrickson et al. (2000), stress levels were raised by informing participants that there was a 50% chance that they would have to deliver a prepared speech, which would be closely evaluated. Not long after receiving this news, all participants were informed that they were lucky and did not have to deliver the speech after all. Participants were then divided into four groups. Two groups watched a movie eliciting positive emotions (contentment and amusement), one group viewed a neutral movie, and one group was exposed to a movie inducing negative emotions (sadness). Rate of recovery from the stress induced by the threat of having to give a speech was measured by registering participants' cardiovascular changes throughout the whole experimental procedure. It was found that participants who were exposed to films that evoked contentment and amusement showed faster cardiovascular recovery than those who watched the neutral or sad films.

These findings support the *undo hypothesis*, demonstrating that positive emotions can speed cardiovascular recovery from the negative emotions induced by being told they had to deliver a speech (see also Fredrickson & Levenson, 1998). This is also another clear example of how our emotional states directly affect our physiological functions. And if negative emotional states persist, disease and physical pathologies can develop as described earlier.

Case study: Public speaking

I was terrified of public speaking up until my late 20s! I even avoided giving speeches at the two weddings at which I was best man. The grooms, who were my very considerate, close mates, gave me permission to just read out the messages of congratulation from those who couldn't be there. Previously, I had also got out of giving presentations in tutorials at university; I just gave short, sharp comments, contributing briefly every now and then, and somehow snuck through. However, my need to be heard became too strong to allow me to go on like this! There were two things that inspired and enabled me to finally take the plunge and give a public talk. Firstly, after returning to studies in naturopathy I realised that if I was ever going to make a living from something that I had such a clear passion for, I would need to get 'out there' and give some talks, and scarily, even lectures. The idea of having a successful private practice certainly instilled in me many *positive emotions*. Secondly, I came across a reference to how Garlic flower essence had helped someone overcome 'crippling' anticipatory anxiety, so I was compelled to investigate further.

Flower essence for anticipatory anxiety: Garlic (FES Group)

In my description of the beneficial qualities of Garlic flower essence (Wells, *Essential Flower Essence Book* p. 197), I allude to the connection between many intense fears in everyday life and our subconscious fear of death: The strengthening and protective qualities of Garlic flower essence do not come from rigid shielding or denial but rather by enabling us to understand and be less fearful about the subtle dimensions in which our life is embedded. It helps us to become comfortable in all our 'skins'! Rudolf Steiner spoke of the parallel spiritual dimension and how we have learned to filter it out of our awareness in order to go about our daily lives. Garlic flower essence enables us to develop a comfortable and secure 'sense,' mainly subconsciously, of the 'other side' of death and beyond, without developing fears and distracting us from our everyday business.

Taking Garlic flower essence certainly was a significant help to me when giving my first public talks. It took the edge off my fear by enabling me to remain *positive* and upbeat in the lead up to speaking. It also helped me hugely at the time of delivering presentations by protecting me from, and minimising my susceptibility to the often highly charged atmosphere of the public arena. Being a highly sensitive person (HSP), I am innately highly susceptible to 'atmosphere.' This flower essence proved to be profoundly beneficial for me.

Negative state
Over-susceptible to negative and highly charged environments
Debilitating sense of foreboding; anticipatory anxiety

Positive state
Vitality, multi-level natural immunity; dynamic protection
Confident, good humoured and 'tuned in' positivity
(Wells, *Essential Flower Essence Book* p. 197)

In a nine-week study by Fredrickson et al. (2008), half of the participants were asked to practise loving kindness meditation (LKM) for nine weeks. This form of meditation is a technique used to increase feelings of warmth and care for self and others, directly evoking positive emotions such as love, contentment, and compassion. The results showed that engaging in LKM resulted in an increase in daily experiences of positive emotions over time. 'The mindful way … is to just observe emotional states impartially, be present, and exercise a moment-to-moment choice of which [positive] emotions to embrace, and which [negatives ones] to let go' (McKenzie & Hassed, 2012, p. 46). Although over the span of nine weeks the increase in positive emotions was not large in magnitude, it was linked to increases in a variety of personal resources, including better mindful attention, self-acceptance, positive relations with others, and good physical health.

Positive emotions can undo the maladaptive effects of a negative emotional experience and also increase our personal capacity to better adapt and manage life experiences. Later I will demonstrate how the *broadening and undoing effect* of positive emotions is an integral part of emotion-focused therapies such as flower essence therapy (FET), meditation therapy, emotion-focused therapy (EFT), and humour therapy, and how it can be applied in recovery from severe and incapacitating types of emotional trauma.

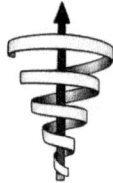

EMOTIONAL INTELLIGENCE

E motional intelligence (EI) is a measure of our ability to be aware of, understand and manage emotions in self and others. Individuals who score highly on emotional intelligence tend to be better able to handle everyday stress, foster a greater number of meaningful close relationships, and be more socially competent in general (see Zeidner et al., 2009, for a review). These individuals are more likely to experience higher levels of wellbeing, or as Ryan & Deci (2001) describe it, 'optimal psychological functioning and experience' (p. 142). EI also helps physical and mental health practitioners to develop and establish better rapport with clients—arguably the most important factor in any effective therapeutic relationship.

DIMENSIONS OF EMOTIONAL INTELLIGENCE

According to Davies et al. (1998), EI has four dimensions:
1. *Noticing and understanding emotions in oneself.*
2. *Noticing and understanding emotions in others.*
3. *Effective regulation of emotion in oneself.*
4. *Using emotions to facilitate performance.*

1st dimension of EI: Noticing our own emotions

The first dimension of EI involves the ability to understand one's deep emotions and be able to express them naturally. A person with high ability in this area will have:

- self-awareness of emotions, thoughts and physical sensations—a well-developed *interoceptive* ability
- the ability to sense, acknowledge and allow emotions to be present and attended to
- the ability to name emotions; broad emotional vocabulary

Emotional awareness is the skill that is perhaps most fundamental to emotional intelligence (Lane, 2000). It is the ability to accurately answer the question: How am I feeling right now? In meditation, you practise remaining in the NOW. While being fully present and experiencing *calm, natural ease and stillness within*, you can attend to and experience a more mindful awareness of all your senses, including your feelings.

Flower essence therapy enables greater emotional awareness and can also help one discern the *primary emotions* that may exist underneath current secondary maladaptive emotional responses and behaviours.

The sailboat: Let's use a sailing analogy. Having a high level of emotional awareness is like having a captain who is able to check the boat's compass regularly during a journey. A captain who devotes sufficient attention to the compass is able to use its feedback to gain information about the current course of the boat. The compass is the most important tool for determining the boat's future direction. A captain who does not pay sufficient attention to the compass or even ignores it is likely to feel lost. In a similar vein, people who are unable to connect to their emotions miss the *inner guide* that provides invaluable information about the comings and goings of the outer world (Gandhiplein 16).

How to better feel emotion

Many of us are confused about how we actually *feel emotions*, let alone how to properly 'read' and interpret them. As mentioned already, each society has its own spoken and unspoken rules about which emotions may be acknowledged and expressed, and also when and where they may be expressed—and these rules are different for each gender! And then there is one's family 'society' which makes its own set of judgments about these things. These influences conspire to inhibit our genuine expression of primary emotions. But there is more to contend with! In this day and age, probably the most common way we modify or disconnect from our emotions is by *dissociating*, being not fully in our bodies, remaining on 'auto-pilot' and going about our everyday business like 'walking heads.' We dissociate from our feelings as a way of coping with stressful situations such as the constant barrage from other people and the media, and the demand to keep pace with life in the fast lane. Is there a better way to cope with going to the supermarket on a busy Saturday morning than disconnecting and dissociating from your emotional reaction to the highly charged environment? Just don't go, or pick a quieter time! For many people, because of past traumatic experiences, dissociating is a way to avoid being emotionally triggered. When we dissociate we are unable to feel or sense, let alone embrace, our primary emotions, and this dramatically inhibits our depth of experience of life, and how we make sense of it. We need to reconnect and better *feel* our emotions because they are fundamental contributors to the way we process the information we receive from the world.

Mindful pauses help us to get in touch with our emotions

When we are aware of our current state of being, we can better identify when a feeling arises. This can be done by noticing our mood, thoughts, and bodily sensations at any given moment, being curious and accepting without judgement whatever emotions/sensations arise. Mindfulness is a natural side-benefit of meditation but you can become immediately more mindful just by pausing to notice the falling leaves of a tree, or listening to the sound of birds outside your window—allowing yourself to stop and smell the roses. It is not about doing anything, it's about stopping, being *still*, noticing, and *feeling*. When you *stop* for a mindful pause—even just for two or three minutes—if you close your eyes it can help you to direct your attention inwards and *look in* for yourself. You will increase your emotional self-awareness by introducing mindful pauses three to five times throughout the day. By interrupting, even briefly, the activity at hand, you connect with the present moment and can reflect on the following questions: What am I feeling now? What kinds of thoughts are present? What can I feel in my body? When communicating about emotions, it is advisable to use language that supports observation: 'In my body, I notice … I am having the thought that …' etc. Many years ago (back in the 80s!) during a course designed for personal growth, the facilitator made a recommendation to a gentleman who found it difficult to connect with his feelings and even more difficult to describe them: 'When you are at home, *every time* you walk from one room to another I want you to stop, close your eyes and ask yourself: How do I feel now?' The man, who happened to own a big house with lots of rooms, reported back the next week: 'Well, the first emotion I felt after walking between a few rooms was one of being pissed off about having to keep doing this! But that's a start I suppose! I persisted and, over time, it certainly raised my general self-awareness. That can only be good, can't it?'

Step 1: STOP what you are doing! Take a seat. Take a few slow, deep breaths, preferably with your eyes closed.

Step 2: Bring your focus inwards and just notice your breathing, then scan your body and notice any tension or other discomfort—for example a sense of urgency to get back to what you were doing. That's OK. Whatever you are feeling is OK. Whatever you are thinking is OK. Be curious and see if any of these feelings, thoughts or sensations in your body begin to change.

Step 3: Notice whether or not your breathing has changed in the last few minutes—either way is OK. Just make the observation, then slowly open your eyes. (OR continue for a while longer, observing your breath while it finds its own natural rhythm, and becomes slower and deeper.)

Meditation, flower essences, and self-regulation

Our ability to effectively regulate our emotions and make behavioural changes is based on the feedback that emotions give us. Restoring our connection with emotions is therefore often a crucial first step in personal growth and/or therapy. Awareness of emotions unveils essential information about our life. Instead of *looking out* for ourselves, we need to *look in* for ourselves. Taking flower essences commonly helps us to *feel better* by helping us to *feel* our emotions *better*. After taking an appropriate flower essence my clients often report an initial increase in awareness of their emotions as well as feeling better in themselves. This recognition/acceptance of an emotion and the information it reveals to them is an essential and efficient way of processing emotions that may previously have been too overwhelming and/or suppressed.

Flower essence for awareness of deep emotion: Fuchsia (FES group)

Fuchsia flower essence has the ability to ground people and allow them to embrace their true feelings. Taking Fuchsia will not unleash painful emotions indiscriminately from the unconscious into an already vulnerable psyche. What it can provide is an inner freedom to make emotional choices from a position of greater awareness.

A friend who relied heavily on daily, strenuous, physical workouts as his only means of dealing with stress came to see me after suffering an injury he knew would incapacitate him for a long time. It was part of his journey as an athlete facing the inevitable processes of ageing. After consideration, we decided Fuchsia flower essence would be helpful. Its effect was to help him to react with greater awareness and in a more grounded and constructive manner to mental and emotional stresses as they occurred at his business and in his everyday life. His stress levels didn't build to the same degree, giving him more freedom of choice about whether he needed to work out or not and how intensely. He still exercises regularly, but now he does so mainly for pleasure and with obvious health benefits, rather than feeling driven to do it.

Negative state
Psychosomatic symptoms resulting from emotional repression (FES)
'False states of emotionality' (FES); disproportionate reactions

Positive state
Deep awareness/Self-understanding
Genuine emotional expression
(Wells, *Essential Flower Essence Book* pp. 182–83)

> A man who has not passed through the inferno of his passions has never overcome them … Whenever we give up, leave behind, and forget too much, there is the danger that the things we have neglected will return with added force. (C.G. Jung, *CW* pp. 275–77)

Identifying emotion fully—interoception

As mentioned, many of us wander around like 'walking heads.' We have lost contact with our inner world—our genuine 'felt' sense. Many of us are unaware of what is going on within ourselves at an emotional level and are therefore mindlessly unperceptive rather than mindfully perceptive of what we are experiencing at any given moment. Our felt sense or interoception involves bi-directional communication between bodily sensation and multiple cognitive centres in the brain. This supports physical and emotional wellbeing, including effective responses to stress via emotional awareness and regulation (Critchley & Garfinkel, 2017). Sensations from the body underlie most if not all of our emotional feelings, particularly those that are most intense and most basic to survival (Craig, 2002). Interoception has a role in survival, supporting regulated responses to sensations that relate to bodily integrity (e.g. sensations of hunger, temperature, and pain) as well as emotional sensations directed at social integration (e.g. positive emotion, affection, and intimacy) and physical survival (e.g. fear and anger/aggression). Interoceptive awareness—the ability to identify, access, understand, and respond appropriately to the patterns of internal signals—provides us with a distinct advantage when responding to life's challenges and making ongoing adjustments (Craig, 2015). In my book, *Embracing the Gift of High Sensitivity* (2021), I speak at length about the capacity for interoception in humans and how well developed it is in highly sensitive individuals, who are also recognised as possessing high emotional intelligence:

> In higher animals (including humans) comes the capacity for interoception—the conscious detection and perception of sensory signals within the body and on the skin, in response to both internal (e.g. 'I'm hungry!') and external stimuli ('What's that noise?'). This is a form of perception that can be so highly developed it is sometimes referred to as a sixth sense. It is not accidental that we often use the words 'feeling' and 'emotion' interchangeably; most often, interoceptive signals are processed as sensations, but sensations are the foundation of our emotional experience, what we feel, even if we are not always fully conscious of them. (p. 19)

Emotional awareness requires an individual to pay attention to the physical sensations (from inside and outside), as well as the thoughts and action tendencies that accompany emotion. Emotional awareness also involves the ability to discern the intensity of an emotion (Frijda, 2007). When we talk about our emotions, we not only describe their nature but also their intensity or duration. For example we might say: 'I woke up this morning feeling really sad. It wasn't until the afternoon that the dark cloud seemed to lift, and I started to feel a bit brighter.'

Intensity of emotions

Sonnemans and Frijda (1994) describe five factors that determine the intensity of emotions:

- **Duration:** How long does the emotion last? What is its onset and when does it reach its peak?
- **Bodily changes:** What are the perceived bodily changes associated with the emotion? What is their magnitude? (Interoceptive awareness is especially important here.)
- **Re-experience:** How often do you recollect the emotional episode in your mind? Do you re-experience the emotion when it is recalled and how strongly?
- **Action tendency:** How strong and severe are the action tendencies associated with the emotion? (E.g. the impulse to kill someone is obviously more severe than just yelling at them; embracing someone is a stronger show of affection than just shaking hands.)
- **Long-term behaviour:** To what extent have emotions and associated events changed your opinion or feelings towards certain things, people and/or yourself? To what extent did the emotion and the events change your long-term behaviour?

We have described earlier in the book how people's inability to identify underlying (primary) emotions and act upon them is associated with a variety of maladaptive emotions and behaviours. These include impulsive binge drinking or eating, inappropriate aggressive responses, and even self-harm. On the other hand, if people do have the ability to identify primary emotions, this awareness can provide them with information about their environment and how they are progressing (or not) towards their goals. This will then positively influence their judgments, decisions, priorities, and how they act upon their feelings/emotions. The ability to attend to and identify one's own emotions is therefore an important prerequisite for using that emotional information in an adaptive way.

Meditation and flower essences in interoception

In order to identify emotions, firstly one must *pay attention to them and allow them to remain in one's consciousness*. So how can we do that? Meditation is a prime enabler of this ability. Rather than avoiding emotions, meditation involves a willingness to allow them to be present and attended to. Our state of *calm, natural ease and stillness within*, reached through meditation practice, enables us to approach our emotions with curiosity and acceptance so that we can say: 'It is absolutely OK for me to experience whatever I experience.' This allows for close self-observation without judgment or attempts to control or change the experience.

We understand that if we pay *no* attention to our emotions it becomes a problem but if we pay *too much* attention to them, that also becomes problematic. Past research has repeatedly shown that *both avoidance and over-engagement with emotions are associated with poor psychological and health outcomes* (Gross, 2002; Salovey et al., 2000; Segerstrom et al., 2003).

Mindfulness meditation practice, by contrast to over-engagement in which the individual becomes completely absorbed or 'possessed' by an emotion, cultivates a safe observational distance from emotion so that you are 'dis-possessed' of it. This distanced or 'decentred' relationship helps the individual to recognise the transient nature of emotions, which come and go 'like clouds in the sky'—a commonly used image in mindfulness practice. We can engage with them, without either avoiding or becoming entangled and over-engaged. In flower essence therapy clients often report similar experiences of decentring, saying things like: 'I was able to step back from the situation, notice how I was feeling, and then make better decisions about what I should do.' They were able to disentangle themselves from their emotions and make decisions from this dis-possessed standpoint rather than responding in a habitual or impulsive and unconscious way, as if possessed by emotion.

Developing the ability to allow emotions to be present may take time and, in some cases, requires caution. Welcoming difficult emotions can be very challenging, especially for people who have previously coped by using avoidance-based strategies such as suppression or disassociation to deal (or *not* deal) with negative affect. This is often the case when people have grown up in environments that disapproved of expressing certain emotions. Or worse, they may have lived in a violent environment in which expression of emotion could put them in physical danger. Many clients (and some friends) have said to me over the years: 'When I was a child I had to walk on eggshells at home to avoid getting into trouble.'

The mere thought of allowing habitually suppressed emotions to be present can trigger fear or panic for many. This fear is often related to the belief that they will not be able to handle the external (life-threatening) consequences, or that they will feel completely overwhelmed by the internal consequences if they give full rein to their emotions. Moreover, with depression and borderline personality disorder, focusing on and staying with negative emotions can overwhelm the client and trigger strong avoidance and disengagement, and even self-harm in some.

When teaching meditation, especially in clinical practice, it is of primary importance for the teacher or therapist to carefully assess a client's abilities to allow negative emotions, or whatever else may emerge, to be present. For some clients—in my experience a small minority—it can be helpful to adopt a slow, step-by-step desensitising approach to their strong, potentially overwhelming emotions. A therapist who has already established a relationship of trust with their client can allow an individual to experience (or be exposed to) their strong emotions very briefly, initially just by talking about them. And then slowly, the time allowed for emotions to remain present increases (see also my example of mindfulness meditation for chronic pain earlier). In time a client will find that it is possible to experience and observe emotions without being overwhelmed or carried away by them. This will strengthen the client's sense of self-efficacy and belief that they are able to deal with emotions by turning toward rather than away from them.

Flower essence for communication: Scarlet Monkeyflower (FES group)

I utilised FET with a man who was having some difficulty acknowledging and expressing his true feelings to his wife. Their discussions would often become heated—his wife expressed anger and frustration with ease while he, as a response, would become more and more detached, saying things like: 'Be rational. I'll speak to you when you can settle down.' These passive-aggressive comments predictably only aggravated the situation, acting as provocation. His wife could express her intense feelings, but he couldn't, and the situation frightened him. (A lot of his behaviour stemmed from childhood and the repressive environment he was brought up in.)

Looking at the dynamic of their relationship, my client's wife was expressing emotion not only for herself but also for him. The usual outcome was that she was left infuriated, while he just walked away in silence, and nothing got resolved. At other times, however, he would 'out of the blue' express disproportionate anger and frustration over trivial things. Unable to keep a permanently tight lid on his own anger and frustration, his rage would suddenly erupt in response to seemingly random incidents, and then in a flash the anger was gone as quickly as it had appeared.

I prescribed Scarlet Monkeyflower flower essence for him. Over the weeks, he began to feel more comfortable with his feeling responses and, as a consequence, less intimidated by his wife's ability to express them wholeheartedly! He also became better at articulating what he felt and his wife became less frustrated because she no longer had to deal with detached non-responses. I asked him how his wife responded when he overtly expressed some anger and frustration during their 'discussions.' He replied, with a wry smile, 'She initially just looked at me open-mouthed, as if she was in shock!' The new dynamic created between them helped her to remain calmer during their discussions, as she was no longer required to do all the heavy lifting when it came to expressing emotion. Those discussions would now no longer come to an abrupt finish, even if they still became a little heated at times, and they proved to be very productive. The couple became more able to fully engage and relate to each other, which had a flow-on, positive effect on all aspects of their relationship.

Negative state
Sudden, disproportionate anger surges/outbursts
Repressed anger/passion (FES)

Positive state
'Clear communication of deep feelings' (FES)
Genuine passion and emotional spontaneity
(Wells, *Essential Flower Essence Book* p. 304)

There are of course situations where avoidance of emotional expression is required and can even be entirely appropriate. If a person only occasionally avoids experiencing their emotions fully, perhaps for reasons of discretion or because of time constraints, this is not necessarily harmful. For example, if someone is unhappy because their boss consistently treats them unfairly and inappropriately, it probably won't be helpful to tell the boss exactly how they feel at the time an incident occurs, when their anger and frustration is at its most intense. It would be better to wait until the heat of the moment has passed, then return to the issue later and work out a productive strategy for giving tactful feedback. To give another example, if you receive a phone call with upsetting news just before entering a meeting at work, you might distract yourself by focusing on the meeting for the time being. This distraction temporarily reduces your worries and later, at home, you can decide to pay attention to feelings and emotions connected to the news. Another good example of how a balanced mixture of emotional avoidance and expression may work for some people is when one has experienced loss. Responses vary from one person to another and there is no right or wrong way to grieve. Some people publicly express their grief at the time of loss, whereas others may do the opposite, going straight back to work, performing their duties between 9 and 5, and then going home to grieve in their way, with partner, family or even alone. They are not necessarily avoiding or in denial of their grief, they are just allowing these deep emotions to be felt fully at the times when it feels safe and possible to allow themselves to be vulnerable.

In summary, avoidance of emotions is most problematic when the strategy is used as a default way to block experiences on a permanent basis. This is when it can harm relationships and health (see also the section on repressed emotion in physical illness).

2nd dimension of EI: Noticing and understanding emotions in others

The second dimension of EI relates to the ability to perceive and understand emotions in other people. A person with high ability in this area will have:

- awareness and understanding of emotional signs in others
- the ability to infer emotions from verbal and nonverbal signs (e.g. body language, facial expressions etc.)
- the ability to display *empathy*—an essential element of high EI

Studies have shown that the ability to correctly perceive and understand other people's emotions is associated with better personal and social effectiveness. For instance, sensitivity to nonverbal cues and facial expressions in particular, has been associated with better academic performance (e.g. Halberstadt et al. 2001; Nowicki & Duke, 1994). Moreover, even at a very young age, the ability to read emotions predicts social and academic outcomes years later (Izard et al., 2001). In a clinical context, difficulties in facial emotion recognition have been associated with a range of psychiatric disorders, including depression (e.g. Surguladze et al., 2004), schizophrenia (e.g. Kohler et al., 2010), autism (e.g. Humphreys et al., 2007), and borderline personality disorder (e.g. Domes et al., 2009). These findings support the notion that the ability to recognise emotions in other people is an important aspect of optimal human functioning. Past research has provided strong evidence that humans universally recognise the facial expressions of seven emotions:

anger, contempt, disgust, fear, joy, sadness, and surprise (Elfenbein & Ambady, 2002). Further findings suggest that people more accurately recognise emotions expressed by members of their own nationality, ethnicity, or region (Elfenbein & Ambady, 2002), as there are subtle differences across cultural groups.

Fieldman Barrett (2017) provides good evidence for a perspective that, although it doesn't completely contradict the above, certainly adds another consideration when we are assessing an individual's perception of emotions in others. She puts forward a convincing case that *'we all construct perceptions of each other's emotions* [and we perceive others as happy, sad, or angry] *by applying our own emotion concepts to what we see. ...* We simulate with such speed that emotion concepts work in stealth, and it seems to us as if emotions are broadcast from the face, voice, or any other part [of the person], and we merely detect them' (p. 51). This concept that we do at least to some degree construct our perceptions of each other's emotions, indicates that we can influence our reality by influencing how we 'see' and react to our world and people in it. There have been times when I have felt apprehensive about pointing something out to a person when I thought they might react negatively—for example with my kids over the years! Because I have already constructed their hostile response in my mind, a tense exchange becomes more likely. I believe this is another significant area in which FET and meditation can have a strong positive influence on how we experience and interpret our world and the emotions expressed by those around us.

FE therapy, meditation, and perception of emotion in others

FET and meditation enable us to *re*-construct (or *re*-vision) our perception of the world and others in a positive way. Other people (and the world) then respond better. When I am positive in my general outlook, people are more likely to respond to me in a positive way.

When speaking about Oregon Grape flower essence, Kaminski and Katz (FES) tell us that some people 'fear the worst in terms of emotional hostility from those nearby and may be paranoid about how people around will react [to them] ... [When] these patterns were learned in childhood from the family or culture, and have not been healed,' individuals are set up to expect the world to be hostile, unfair and unsafe. This fear can become a self-fulfilling prophecy—we look for ill will in the world and that is what we find, and this cycle of alienation can leave us with a tendency to avoid full involvement (Wells, *Essential Flower Essence Book* p. 266).

Flower essence for withdrawing projection: Oregon Grape (FES group)

Oregon Grape is an excellent example of a flower essence that can help us *re-construct perceptions of each other's emotions* and step forward confidently without projecting our own internal fears onto others.

Negative state
Socially paranoid (FES)
Fear-driven defensiveness which can ostracise others

Positive state
Trusting others' goodwill (FES)
Inclusiveness (FES)

Daily meditation practice has been shown to produce measurable changes in brain regions associated with memory, sense of self, empathy, and stress. Studies have even documented changes in the brain's grey matter over time. These changes alter for the better our perception of the world, ourselves and others. Because of the brain's capacity for neuroplasticity, meditation can literally rewire established, maladaptive neurological pathways/circuits set up in childhood and/or induced by trauma, and create more adaptive ones.

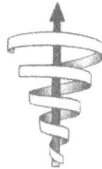

EMOTIONAL EXPRESSION

Nonverbal elements that accompany the spoken word are at least as important as the actual words themselves in creating meaning. Body language comprises 'the conscious and unconscious movements and postures by which attitudes and feelings are communicated' (*Oxford English Dictionary*). This can include micro-expressions, posture, stance, proxemics (sense of personal space), kinesics (gestures), eye contact, speech style, and speech tone. People with high EI are more attuned to these subtle signals. The ability to accurately decipher emotional expressions plays a key role in social interaction (Kilts et al., 2003) as it facilitates appropriate responses and bonding (Isaacowitz et al., 2007). There are different ways to 'read' other people's emotions, including paying attention to speech (i.e. vocal inflections, tone of voice, word use), body movements and facial expressions.

Three different forms of emotional expression

VERBAL expression:
EMOTIONAL WORDS: e.g. 'I'm angry'
METAPHORS: e.g. 'I feel trapped'
PITCH: high/low
LOUDNESS: high/low
RATE OF SPEECH: slow/fast

NONVERBAL expression

Facial expressions:
EYES: open, upper/lower white showing
EYELID: raised, tense, drawn up
EYEBROWS: raised, lowered curved, drawn together
NOSTRILS: flared
MOUTH: open, closed, corners up, corners down
LIPS: tensed, relaxed, stretched, drawn back

Body movements
HEAD: tilted up/down, turning away
MOVEMENT: fast/slow
CHEST: expanded
SHOULDERS: back, slumped
ARMS: limp at sides, up
HANDS: covering face, holding head, clapping

Speech

People use thousands of terms to *verbally* express a wide variety of emotional states (Russell, 1991; Sabini & Silver, 2005). Often the words that are used point directly to the emotion experienced. For instance, the experience of fear may be expressed by saying 'I am afraid.' Likewise, experiencing sadness may be communicated by stating 'I feel sad.' The intensity of an emotion can also be expressed through words: 'I'm scared *witless!*' In addition, people often use figurative expressions to express how they feel, rather than directly naming an emotional state. Figurative expressions rely on metaphors or analogies to express subjective experiences. In the English language, there are many expressions that are commonly used to talk about emotions. For example, people may say they 'tremble like a leaf,' 'feel trapped' or 'hit a low.' Emotions are also expressed by *nonverbal* qualities of speech such as pitch, volume, and rate of speech. For example, in a situation where it is unacceptable to directly state that one is angry—in public, for instance—pitch, volume and rate of speech may be used to convey anger.

Facial expressions

The face is a dynamic canvas on which people display their emotional states, and we use others' facial expressions to decode these states (e.g. Willis & Todorov, 2006). For instance, a person who is surprised may raise their eyebrows, open their eyes wide, and drop their jaw. These expressions have been referred to as macro-expressions and are relatively easy to detect; they take place when people do not try to conceal their emotions. Macro-expressions often occur when people are alone or with close others such as family and friends. Micro-expressions, on the other hand, occur in a fraction of a second, sometimes as fast as 1/30 of a second. Because of their speed, they are more difficult to detect. Micro-expressions can take place when an individual is trying to conceal emotion. For example, a person who tries to hide anger in response to a snide remark may very briefly press their lips firmly together (immediate angry reaction) but quickly cover this by smiling.

Bodily expressions

There is lots of evidence that numerous emotions, including pride, shame, anger, fear, and disgust (e.g. de Gelder et al., 2011; Keltner, 1995; Tracy et al., 2009) can be discerned in nonverbal bodily displays. Pride, for instance, is typically signalled by an expanded chest, upward head tilt, and arms either spread out from the body or with hands on hips or fists raised overhead (Tracy & Matsumoto, 2008; Tracy & Robins, 2004). Past research has identified consistent bodily expressions for joy, happiness, pride, shame and embarrassment, fear, anger, disgust, and sadness (see Witkower & Tracy, 2018 for a review). I believe this is just another example of 'the message in the body.'

Synergy

When I give a lecture or make a video or podcast, I love to use hand gestures as I speak. I feel more comfortable that way, and I believe that for the most part these gestures enhance and act in synergy with the words and other modes of expression I am using to convey my point. And further, I feel hamstrung and inhibited if I cannot move around and gesture while I am lecturing. Many scholars agree with me that facial, bodily, and verbal expressions of emotions work synergistically together. For instance, Jorgensen (1998) argues that 'in essence, by focusing on one element (i.e. verbal) of the emotional appeal to the exclusion of the other dimensions of the message (i.e. nonverbal), researchers are no longer studying valid communication processes, but rather disassociated parts of the whole' (p. 407). Focusing on words alone, as we are often forced to do in emails and texts for instance, makes it very difficult to decode the emotions of another person accurately. Nonverbal cues can modify, augment, illustrate, accentuate, and contradict the words they accompany (Burgoon & Buller, 1994). I feel sure this is why the use of emojis has become so prevalent. They enable a person to compensate for the lost emotional dimension when communicating using words alone. (However, like hand gestures and body movements, emojis can sometimes be overdone to the point that they become a distraction from what someone is actually trying to say.) Research findings suggest that faces and bodies are perceived holistically, and information is perceptually integrated (Aviezer et al., 2012; Meeren et al., 2005).

Two examples of synergistic facial, bodily, and verbal expressions of emotion

JOY: *Bodily expression:*

- head tilted up
- chest out
- arms out
- upwards movement
- fast, energetic movement

Facial expression:

- raised cheeks
- crow's feet near the outside of the eyes
- corners of the lips drawn back and up
- teeth exposed

Verbal expression:

- increased pitch of speech
- increased loudness of speech
- increased rate of speech

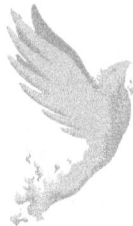

ANGER: *Bodily expression:*
- head tilted down
- arms forward
- fists clenched
- hitting motions
- leaning forward
- stamping feet
- fast movement

Facial expression:
- tensed lower eyelid
- bulging eyes
- firmly pressed lips
- corners of lips down
- flared nostrils
- lower jaw jutting out

Verbal expression:
- increased pitch of speech
- increased loudness of speech
- increased rate of speech

We can extract emotional information from carefully observing another person's verbal and nonverbal behaviours. But whatever the situation, the better a person can read their own feelings, the better they will be able to read another's.

Transference

When thinking about our perceptions of others' emotions, we should also be aware of the process of *transference*, which is a factor in all relationships, though the term itself is mainly used in psychotherapy. Transference occurs when a person unknowingly transfers feelings about someone from their past onto another. A simple and common example may be when a person projects the feelings they have had for one of their parents onto someone else, as when a younger woman projects her feelings for her father onto an older male at work who subconsciously reminds her of her father.

Unconscious feelings such as these can become very deep and intense, especially between a therapist and a client, and give rise to countertransference, which is essentially the reverse of transference. In contrast to transference (which is about the client's emotional reaction to the therapist), countertransference can be defined as the therapist's emotional reaction to emotion that has been transferred onto them by the client.

One form of countertransference is when you feel intensely or 'pick up on' an emotion that actually belongs to someone else. For example, you might be talking to someone and you begin to feel anger building in you, but strangely this anger is not felt (initially at least), towards the other person, and has no other cause that you can identify—it doesn't feel as if it 'belongs' to you. Often when this occurs, the person you are speaking with is, in fact, angry about something but is not displaying it in any overt way.

Emotional boundaries

It should be noted that highly sensitive persons (HSPs) are very susceptible to overt and covert feelings generated by others, because of a normal human trait (*not* a pathological condition) known as Sensory Processing Sensitivity. It is now believed that HSPs make up around a third of the population—a significant minority who generally don't make as much 'noise' as the rest of the less sensitive population. (This portion of the population has an even greater representation in counselling and health care, both as practitioners and among those seeking help.)

HSPs think and feel very deeply and cannot help but notice the nuances of their interactions with others: 'HSPs are keenly aware of the moods and emotions of other people and are readily affected by them, rapidly responding to the slightest stimulus and *gaining much more information than less sensitive people from nonverbal clues*. Genuine empathy— understanding how someone is feeling, and *sharing their emotion*—comes naturally to them' (Wells, *Embracing the Gift of High Sensitivity* p. 41). In one experiment, researchers (Dimitroff et al., 2017) found that around a fifth of those who volunteered to take part in the experiment (which happens to be only marginally less than the proportion of HSPs in the general population) experienced a surge in levels of the stress hormone cortisol just watching other people undergoing a stressful experience. This is called subconscious emotional contagion. Sensory cues provide information about someone else's fear or anger, and a highly sensitive person will be more receptive to this information and will respond— in some cases, as the research showed, deeply enough to affect them physiologically. Emotional contagion is thought to be the basis on which empathy is built.

The research found a strong link between those who are more susceptible to emotional contagion and higher empathy scores. One theory suggests that feelings of empathy might involve a particular kind of brain activity, where nerve cells called *mirror neurons* fire in a certain way when one animal observes another, so that their brain activity 'mirrors' the behaviour of the other. In humans, research has shown that this extends to mirroring the other's feelings/emotions. In a research paper called 'Monkey see, monkey do?: The role of mirror neurons in human behavior' (2011), Arthur Glenberg states that the brain's mirror neuron system plays a role in how we understand other people's speech, how and why we understand other people's actions and even how and why we understand other people's minds and the intentions behind their actions. Emotions are contagious because of mirror neurons in the brain (Wells, *Embracing the Gift of High Sensitivity* p. 42). Hence, when HSP therapists are working with clients, or just relating to others in everyday life, they need to protect themselves by maintaining boundaries, especially those of a more subtle nature, even more than others who are less sensitive.

Flower essence for emotional boundaries: Pink Yarrow (FES group)

I have a strong personal relationship with Pink Yarrow—and no, I don't have deep and meaningfuls with it in my garden, although I do glance at it fondly! It has helped me greatly to protect my highly sensitive nature so that I can embrace it for the gift it is, and utilise it beneficially, both with clients and in my personal life, without it becoming my Achilles' heel! Pink Yarrow acts like an energetic emotional buffer between us and others so that emotional boundaries are better defined. Pink Yarrow flower essence assists people who are emotionally oversensitive and act like 'psychic sponges,' *absorbing everyone else's feelings*. In the negative state we can too easily engage in *'overly sympathetic identification with others'* (Kaminski & Katz, FES) and take on all the problems of partners, family members, colleagues, close friends or clients.

Negative state
Overly sympathetic—'psychic sponge'
Lacking emotional boundaries (FES)

Positive state
'Self-contained consciousness' (FES) while maintaining empathy
Emotional clarity; acknowledging others' feelings without
taking them on yourself
(Wells, *Essential Flower Essence Book* p. 277)

Meditation and emotional boundaries

Practising meditation regularly enables me, when working with clients or just hanging out with other people, to recognise and observe strong emotions without judgement, whether they are projected onto me through transference or just sensed by me. Regularly experiencing *inner calm, natural ease and stillness* in meditation helps us get better and better at observing feelings and thoughts, even uncomfortable ones, with curiosity and acceptance, and without becoming overwhelmed and consumed by them. There are many different forms of *guided meditation* that can help people develop better and healthier emotional boundaries, for example, creating a sense of being surrounded by a protective sphere of white light.

3rd dimension of EI: Emotional self-regulation

The third dimension of EI involves the ability to effectively deal with one's own emotions. Emotional self-regulation helps people cope better, and display resilience and sociability. People with high capability in this respect will be able to:

- choose how to respond to emotions
- think/pause before they act
- separate emotions from logical understanding and have awareness of their emotions' influence on their world view

Emotional self-regulation for coping, resilience and sociability

Emotional regulation refers to an individual's attempt to increase, maintain, or decrease their experience of emotions, positive and negative. Harte (2019, p. 33) states: 'To emotionally regulate is the ability to respond to the ongoing demands of experience with a range of emotions in a manner that is socially tolerable and sufficiently flexible to permit spontaneous reactions as well as the ability to delay spontaneous responses as needed.' This ability to effectively regulate and manage one's emotions is a crucial skill and is associated with positive mental and physical health outcomes (Gross & Muñoz, 1995; Sapolsky, 2007), relationship satisfaction (Murray, 2005), and work performance (Diefendorff et al., 2000).

Being able to regulate your emotions helps you to reach your short-term and long-term goals. I am reminded of the old saying about saving money by managing (self-regulating) the urge to overspend: 'Watch the cents and the dollars will take care of themselves.' Difficult situations may trigger negative emotions such as fear or anger, causing you to procrastinate or get distracted from your goals.

Meditation is a powerful way to become better able to emotionally self-regulate. If you experience a state of *calm, natural ease and stillness within* often enough through regular practice, this state increasingly infiltrates the rest of your life. You remain aware of your emotional reactions of fear, anger etc., but become more able to accept and see them as something separate from yourself, and can go about your everyday business without them negatively impacting you.

Case study: Hypothetical

While George is driving on the freeway, a car swerves towards him. If George is on 'autopilot' and isn't paying attention to information coming in via his 'fear, fight or flight' response, the other car may collide with him. Alternatively, if George is mindful and responds appropriately, he will be able to brake and swerve in time to avoid an accident. However, even if the other car doesn't hit him, if he cannot regulate his ongoing angry response to the situation, it may distract him to the point where he misses his turnoff and ends up late for work, feeling anxious and flustered. It wasn't the 'crazy' driver's behaviour that made George late, it was his own emotionally unregulated reaction to it! FET enables people to better self-regulate emotion. The above situation might have played out differently if George had been taking an appropriate flower essence such as Scarlet Monkeyflower.

Flower essence for Self-regulation: Scarlet Monkeyflower (FES group)

In the unbalanced state, Scarlet Monkeyflower people feel anger and frustration that is often expressed indirectly or in sudden, inappropriate outbursts. They might keep a lid on disturbing emotions until they finally explode in a fit of rage (FES). Afterwards, frightened by the inappropriateness and intensity of their anger and its effect on others, they repress these powerful emotions once more and so the cycle continues (Wells, *Essential Flower Essence Book* p. 304) After taking the flower essence for a time, people in a balanced state are able to clearly communicate deep feelings as they emerge, spontaneously and honestly, and well before suppressed emotion explodes with an intensity that is out of proportion to the situation.

Negative state
Sudden, disproportionate anger surges/outbursts
Repressed anger/passion (FES)

Positive state
Insight and acceptance of powerful emotions
Genuine passion and emotional spontaneity (FES)

Hypothetical—take two!

After using Scarlet Monkeyflower flower essence for a couple of weeks, George again takes appropriate action in response to the dangerous behaviour of the driver in front of him and continues on his way, a bit shaken and angry at what has just occurred, but more accepting and less at the mercy of rage towards the other driver. Feelings of anger and frustration are manageable, and George doesn't take the actions of the careless driver so personally. The situation loses its heat and lo and behold, George remains alert enough to notice his turnoff and arrive on time, relaxed and ready for work, in a positive Scarlet Monkeyflower state of mind. Fuchsia is another flower essence that addresses a person's inability to take opportunities for conscious self-expression due to repression of our true emotional responses. Then the emotional 'charge' associated with all of life's experiences continues to accumulate until the slightest trigger can provoke an extreme reaction in a hyper-emotional release (Wells, *Essential Flower Essence Book* p. 185).

STRATEGIES FOR REGULATING EMOTION

People regulate their emotions in personal relationships and in the workplace to realise goals such as avoiding conflict with others (Parrot, 1993; Tamir, 2009). For example, someone who feels anger towards a co-worker may try to hide their feelings in order to maintain a favourable impression; another person who is feeling sad may try to improve their mood by focusing on things they're grateful for in order to feel better.

When trying to manage emotions we use a range of strategies, some more successful than others, and some more adaptive/positive than others. All of them relate to how we direct our attention—do we direct it *away from negative emotions* by distraction, suppression or dissociation, or do we direct it *towards practices that reduce stress* and so enhance our capacity to deal with difficult situations?

Directing attention away from distress and discomfort

This strategy, known as *attentional regulation using informational bias*, can be effective when used consciously. Examples include:

- During a hard training session at the gym you *counter-regulate by paying attention to information that is in contrast to your current state*, ignoring pain and discomfort to focus on the fitness and strength you are developing and the joy of performing better, while reading the motivational posters around the walls! Once the hard work is done you can *pay attention to information that is in agreement with your current state*—you're hungry and focus on advertisements for delicious-looking food on the way home!
- Thinking pleasurable thoughts and/or creating positive mental images ('eye candy') to avoid feeling stressed, for example by the tedium of a job.

However, other forms of information bias can be quite maladaptive, with negative results in the long term. These include:

- *Suppression and dissociation:* Trying not to think particular thoughts; trying not to show feelings—keeping a stiff upper lip! Ironically, suppression often results in the very emotional outcomes that people set out to avoid. Scarlet Monkeyflower and Fuchsia flower essences are useful in this situation.
- *Distracting oneself* from an emotional experience or trigger, e.g. looking at your phone to avoid the discomfort of being looked at or not knowing how to act.
- *Stress-induced eating* for comfort, to reduce sadness, anger and anxiety in the short term.

Directing attention towards calming the nervous system

Another strategy involves practices that directly address stress and sensitivity to triggers by calming the nervous system. These include:

- *Diaphragmatic breathing:* Deep belly breathing to calm yourself (and your sympathetic nervous system).
- *Progressive muscle relaxation:* Tensing and releasing one muscle group at a time to relax the whole body (and the mind).
- *Time out:* Going for a walk, taking a break to practise deep belly breathing or meditation.
- *Meditation:* Being aware of your emotions in an attentive, curious and non-judgmental way.
- *Acceptance:* Through practices such as meditation, allowing feelings to be present without acting on them because they no longer have the same intense impact.

- *Venting*. Verbally expressing negative emotions, perhaps *exaggerating* what you feel.
- *Expressive writing* about past emotional experiences, including one's thoughts, feelings, and perceptions of events—a positive and adaptive example of venting that enables self-managed *desensitisation and reprocessing* of past trauma.

Many strategies involve a combination of these two approaches.

- *Cognitive reappraisal* reframes or reinterprets a situation in order to down-regulate negative reactions, e.g. if you're feeling depressed because you failed an exam, you remind yourself that you'll have a chance to re-sit, and now you know where you went wrong so you'll do better next time.
- *Cognitive dissonance reduction* tries to resolve an inconsistency between two understandings of a situation. For example, someone enjoys smoking while knowing it is very detrimental to health; they are able to downplay this conflict by noting that aunty is 85 and still smokes, or they say, 'I enjoy smoking, and if I die earlier that's OK!'

We can all get better at learning adaptive self-regulatory skills. Research consistently finds that self-regulation strategies support the drive for lifelong learning by enhancing motivation, enriching our ability to reason and improving performance outcomes (Clark, 2012). Highly resourceful people use a diverse range of emotional self-regulation strategies that help them pursue their goals in daily life. Unfortunately, less resourceful people use only a limited number of self-regulation strategies and are more likely to abandon self-regulation in the face of frustration, resulting in untimely emotional outbursts, impulsive decisions etc. Emotionally intelligent people are highly resourceful because they are able to select and use the most effective self-regulation strategies for the situation.

The process model of emotional regulation

According to the process model of self-regulation (for a review, see Gross & Thompson, 2007), negative/maladaptive emotions develop and go through stages of increasing intensity over time if self-regulation strategies are not used:

Stage 1: A situation (imagined or real) *triggers* an emotion.

Stage 2: The individual *focuses* on this situation in a certain way.

Stage 3: The individual *interprets* the situation in a certain way.

Stage 4: The individual *responds* in a certain way in an attempt to deal with the emotion.

Example

A student fails a practical exam (Stage 1 *trigger*). They focus on the failure, and on the examiner who made the assessment (Stage 2 *focus*). Next, they perceive the result as unfair and feel they have been judged too harshly (Stage 3 *interpretation*), then they try to suppress feelings of anger towards the examiner, not wishing to upset them and attract even harsher judgement (Stage 4 *response*). Emotions increase in intensity as someone progresses through the four stages. Even though the student is able to suppress their anger to some degree, by Stage 4 it is intense and will remain so unless they can modify their interpretation of the original situation.

According to the process model, down-regulation strategies can be applied during any of the four stages (DeSteno et al., 2013), but it is easiest to do this in the earlier stages when emotions are less intense and less entrenched. Using the above example, the student could down-regulate their emotions as early as Stage 2 by shifting their focus away from their sense of injustice and towards respecting the knowledge of the examiner, being receptive to guidance, and learning from the experience to improve future performance. This is a good example of the self-regulatory strategy of *cognitive reappraisal* that focuses on looking at an emotional state or trigger from a different perspective. Gentian flower essence can be very helpful here.

Flower essence for cognitive reappraisal: Gentian (Bach group)

The gentian plant seeks to establish itself on hilltop grassland—this signature relates to how the flower essence helps us gain a *broad perspective on the world* so that we are able to put things in context. Gentian flower essence helps us to face life's challenges with courage, a light heart and a buoyant view. It broadens our perspectives and allows us to see the positive aspects of our situation. We learn to tolerate the ups and downs of life with a resilient, positive and purposeful attitude.

Negative state
Depressed; narrow-minded view of problems
Discouraged by setbacks

Positive state
Ability to *oversee* and understand
Resilient—undeterred by setbacks
(Wells, *Essential Flower Essence Book* pp. 184–85)

In the example given above, the student could also down-regulate emotions at Stage 3 by accepting their anger/frustration, allowing emotions to be present while being less negatively affected by them, and then responding differently (Stage 4) in a more adaptive way. This strategy for regulating emotion focuses on changing the relationship with emotions and becoming more accepting of them.

As I have mentioned previously, meditation, along with acceptance-based coping (a by-product of meditation practice) does not aim to reduce or suppress the intensity of an emotion—it focuses on a person's ability and willingness to allow an emotion to be present, so that they can establish a better relationship with it, resist it less, be less judgmental about it, and become more and more comfortable with its presence. All these changed responses help to diffuse its negative impact by the time Stage 4 is reached. Metaphorically, a person becomes able to balance the experience of anger and frustration with responding and taking appropriate action. Acceptance of feelings also allows for cognitive reappraisal of their initial focus (Stage 2) so that they can choose a more positive one. (It should be noted here that regular practice of meditation makes *acceptance* a part of everyday life, so that in the example given above, the student may not have been *triggered* so easily in the first place (Stage 1). Practising meditation ensures that you don't over-identify with a feeling, as occurs when an emotion 'takes over.' By staying present in the moment, experiencing *calm, natural ease and stillness within,* you are able to better observe emotions with curiosity and without judgment and as something separate from your overall Self. You perceive emotion as transient, something that you can choose to engage with or let go.

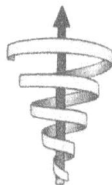

Applying self-regulating strategies

According to the process model of emotional regulation, self-regulatory strategies can be applied at various points throughout the aforementioned four stages:

At Stage 1
Situation selection

Situation selection involves placing yourself in a situation where unwanted emotions are unlikely to be experienced, or desired emotions are likely to be experienced. For example, if you are afraid of being rejected by strangers you might avoid social situations where you meet new people. Likewise, if you wish to experience joy you might decide to hang out with close friends.

Situation modification

Situation modification refers to modifying your immediate environment in a way that allows you to have a more positive emotional response. For example, you might play background music that improves the ambience, or discreetly walk away from an unpleasant conversation, or ensure that at your workplace, you only see a certain person you feel uncomfortable around, within a larger group of colleagues.

At Stage 2
Attentional deployment

Attentional deployment refers to directing your attention in a way that lets you experience a positive emotional response. For example, you might close your eyes when watching a scary or violent scene in a movie (or on the news after being given a trigger warning by the presenter), and you might briefly think about something consoling; or you might avoid a person you don't want to talk to by seeking out someone you do enjoy talking to; or on your day off, you might shift your attention from work problems to things that give you enjoyment and help you relax.

At Stage 3
Cognitive change

Cognitive change involves altering the way you think about things that trigger emotion. By thinking differently about an emotional situation, the *meaning* of the situation can change. In emotion-focused therapy, for instance, one can even reappraise and reframe the memory of a traumatic experience to such an extent that neural pathways laid down in the brain in response to the trauma are reprogrammed. We have already seen an example of this in the student who reappraises an exam failure in light of the opportunity it presents to allow them to re-sit, better prepared. Another example of *cognitive reappraisal* might be realising, after making what you believe was a wrong decision that led to an undesired outcome, 'I have eliminated that option. Now I feel clearer about what I really want and how to get there.'

Case study: Reappraisal

Here is an example from my own life in which I found something to be grateful about when facing a challenging situation. In my mid-twenties, I badly broke my forearm, snapping both of the bones completely while playing Australian Rules football. At the time, I was just getting by financially, receiving a modest income as a football player and making up the shortfall by driving taxis, after leaving a teaching role with the Education Department to study naturopathy full time. Now, with a broken arm, both my sources of income were gone! I was out of action for the rest of the football season, and was unable to drive. My only option was to move back home to my caring and welcoming mother and enjoy free rent and meals for the 6 months of rehab—thanks Mum! I was able not only to continue my studies but also give my full attention to a huge amount of reading on a subject I was passionate about. So, within a very short time I was able to *cognitively reappraise* the situation and *reframe* it as one of the best things that could have happened to me!

Figure 5: My experience of the broadening effect of cognitive reappraisal

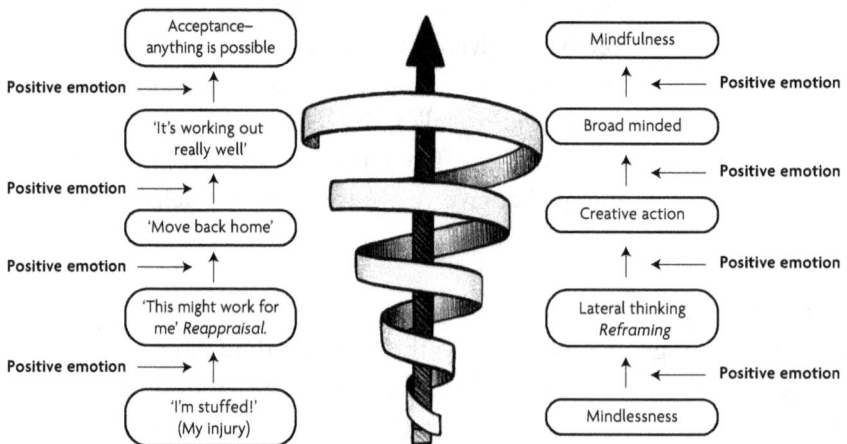

At Stage 4
Response modulation

Response modulation means trying to deal with an emotion once it is fully activated. For example, a person in sales may try to manage anger by using *diaphragmatic breathing* as an emotional self-regulatory strategy when an irritating customer keeps asking the same question. Another example may be when one is able to observe feelings of fear mindfully to prevent oneself from acting upon them: Feel the fear, and do it anyway. These are examples of emotional self-regulatory strategies of *meditation* and *acceptance* which allow feelings to be present without responding negatively or acting out.

Adopting a personal growth mindset

Many of us have used emotional self-regulation strategies to achieve *short-term* goals such as dieting to lose weight so our clothes fit us again, doing regular exercise to prepare for a mini-marathon, or not drinking alcohol in the evening because you need to be clear-headed for a job interview the next day. But often, after achieving short-term goals, we slip back into old patterns of impulsiveness, and the self-regulatory skills we utilised lapse. To learn, maintain and develop a diverse range of sustainable emotional self-regulatory strategies that help us pursue and achieve our *long-term* goals, it is important to adopt a personal growth mindset and develop the aspiration to be a better person overall. This will not only benefit our health and wellbeing but also have a positive impact on those around us. Flower essence therapy, meditation and emotion-focused therapies can play a significant role in developing this mindset, as many client cases throughout this book testify.

The word *flow* has come into use in positive psychology to describe an optimal state of consciousness that becomes more and more accessible as we develop our potential. In a flow state, you're fully immersed in an activity and experiencing intense focus and enjoyment. Achieving flow, as identified by psychologist Mihaly Csikszentmihalyi (2008), occurs when there's a perfect balance between challenge and skill. This state leads to a loss of self-consciousness and a changed sense of time, where hours feel like minutes. By reaching flow, you can boost productivity, enhance creativity, and find deep satisfaction. Understanding and harnessing flow can transform your work and personal life, helping you perform at your best and enjoy the process more fully.

Figure 6: Personal growth mindset—consistent access to flow state arises
when we become unconsciously skilled

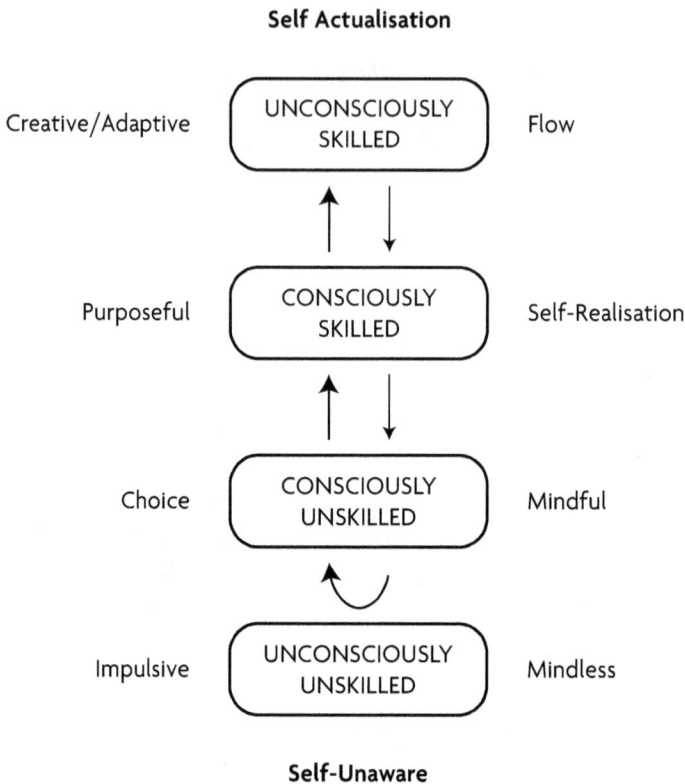

Self Actualisation

Creative/Adaptive	UNCONSCIOUSLY SKILLED	Flow
Purposeful	CONSCIOUSLY SKILLED	Self-Realisation
Choice	CONSCIOUSLY UNSKILLED	Mindful
Impulsive	UNCONSCIOUSLY UNSKILLED	Mindless

Self-Unaware

Flow expert Csikszentmihalyi describes seven characterisitics of
people in the flow state:

- Individuals believe they can achieve the task at hand, and have
  reached a *consciously skilled* level in regard to the task.
- They are *mindful* and can concentrate on the task.
- They are *purposeful* and can concentrate on clear goals.
- They can receive immediate feedback and have *choices.*
- They can act with deep and effortless *creative, adaptive*
  involvement that allows them to rise above frustrations.
- They are unconsciously skilled enough to experience a sense
  of control over their own actions.
- They can lose all sense of self in a task, but then, once the
  task is completed, they can experience a stronger sense of self,
  because they have reached a level of *self-realisation.*

BROADENING & UNDOING

Now we will look at the broadening and undoing effects of positive emotions on recovery from and better management of severe emotional trauma and stress, using therapies such as meditation, flower essence therapy (FET), emotion-focused therapy (EFT), and humour therapy.

POSITIVE EMOTIONS AS THERAPY
Meditation

Meditation practice helps us to 'zoom out' from within, broadening our perspective on our thoughts and feelings by viewing them within a far bigger context, provided by an all-pervading state of *calm, natural ease and stillness.* This particular form of broad awareness 'is intrinsically healing. ... [It is a] present moment awareness that is nonjudging, without agenda, unconditionally accepting' (Rogers, 1980; see also Duncan et al., 2010). This mindshift, in which the individual starts to observe rather than become consumed by their emotion, has also been referred to as *decentring* (Safran & Segal, 1990), cognitive *defusion* (Shapiro & Carlson, 2009) and *deautomatisation* (Deikman, 1982). By taking a step back from the feelings and thoughts associated with an emotion we create room for a different, more mindful and adaptive response rather than the narrow, often impulsive, maladaptive response initially induced when experiencing an emotion. At the same time and on a cellular level this shift enhances the neuroplasticity of the brain, modifying neural pathways that were created in response to emotional trauma, and which lead to maladaptive responses such as panic/anxiety in PTSD sufferers, for instance. Permanent healing of the emotional pain of past trauma becomes possible.

Let's now revisit Figure 2 from earlier in the book (p. 29), which describes the process of grieving, and use it to describe how meditation broadens one's perspective on negative, maladaptive feelings and thoughts associated with trauma. The *expectation* may be that, after a time, the pain of trauma will fade into insignificance. However, the *reality* is that the pain remains, but one's mental perspective can broaden and become more mindful over time, especially through meditation, so that the pain has less and less negative impact overall. Within the broadened experience of the mind (and the associated neural pathway changes in the brain over time), trauma slowly contracts into the background. The person grows and is more and more able to put their pain into the perspective of a life horizon that keeps expanding. I have used FET repeatedly with clients over the years to help them get a better sense of the needs, values, and strengths available within the Self, so as to find deeper meaning and broaden their life perspective. From this awareness, they can make personally responsible decisions that also *feel* deeply right and authentic.

FET for a broadened perspective: Pansy (FES group)

I have often used Pansy flower essence with people who have received a medical diagnosis and are feeling depressed and powerless because they have become resigned to a particular outcome, feeling that there is nothing they can do, and that the worst is inevitable. Pansy flower essence is particularly helpful in modifying the mindset that develops when we become over-identified with our illness.

Pansy has helped many clients regain hope—not false hope!—so that they become positive and open to possibility. Pansy flower essence's beneficial qualities are a great example of the *broadening effect* (Fig. 7), helping people to feel more positive and uplifted. While remaining grounded, their perspective broadens and their minds open up to more proactive choices and potentially more and better outcomes. Pansy flower essence can help us adapt and change our thinking without being blindly influenced by or resigned to the attitudes of the surrounding culture. Just as the plant displays its independent nature in the wild as the first flower to bloom in disturbed ground, so the flower essence can help us to think outside the square and broaden our perspective in relation to health issues (Wells, *Essential Flower Essence Book* p. 267).

Figure 7: Pansy flower essence and the broadening effect

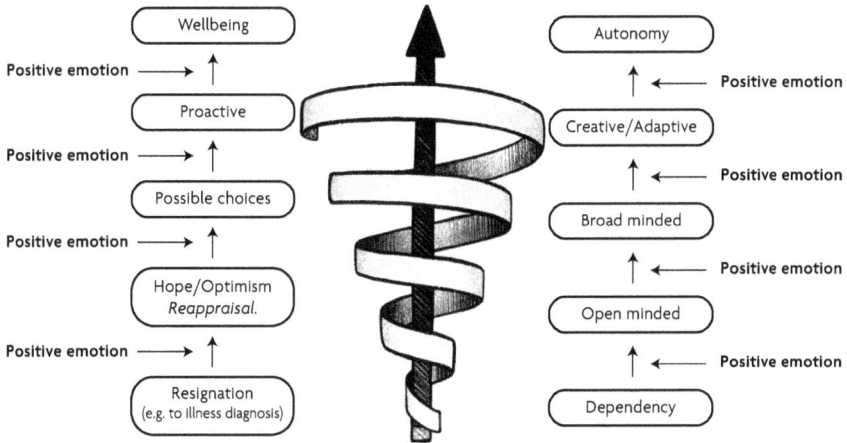

Negative state
Pessimism with reductive/exclusive thinking
A disease model of health

Positive state
Optimism with broad/inclusive thinking
A wellness model of health

The name Pansy comes from the French pensée, or 'thought' and for centuries a gift of pansies has meant, 'You are in my thoughts' in the language of flowers. In other words, I am sending you my best wishes (*positive thoughts*). Pansies can also represent *free-thinking* and the ability to reflect. Often used as a get-well flower, pansies are commonly given to someone who is going through a rough patch to help elevate their mood and lift their spirits (Wells, *Essential Flower Essence Book* p. 267).

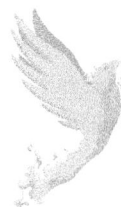

Emotion-Focused Therapy (EFT)

Emotion-focused therapy is an evidence-based treatment for depression, trauma, anxiety, and the effects of abuse, marital or familial distress, and unresolved relationship issues. In EFT, emotions are viewed as providing information about our needs, values, and goals. As a result of past experiences, we may have learned to ignore, dismiss or suppress emotions or avoid unpleasant emotions we fear will cause harm, and thus we lack emotional awareness.

The focus of EFT is to use therapeutic interventions that enable us to connect with, explore, increase awareness, make sense of and transform emotional experiences. Through EFT clients learn how to connect with their feelings in a healthy and adaptive way by increasing their capacity for other positive and/or adaptive emotions. When this becomes possible, they can experience past trauma in a way that lets them feel safer and more empowered. In EFT there are many examples of how introducing positive emotions 'undoes' the maladaptive effects of negative emotions previously experienced during and after trauma. As with meditation and flower essence therapy, emotion-focused therapy can enhance the brain's neuroplasticity in a beneficial way. It can enable neural pathways set up in response to past trauma to change from being maladaptive (leading to anxiety and negative behaviours), to being adaptive and leading to positive behaviours and outcomes.

Let's say a person experienced abuse as a child. Now adult, the individual is aware that their unresolved emotional pain is having a negative impact on their life, and they are committed to working with a therapist to process and heal the trauma. EFT focuses on narrative content (the story a client tells—in this example about their experiences of abuse as a child) and on processing the painful emotions connected to that story, which underlie the presenting problem. As a client's memories of past trauma emerge naturally during consultation, a well-trained therapist can make moment-to-moment decisions about how to proceed with therapy, checking with the client to make sure they are ready to revisit painful experiences. As Melissa Harte (2019) points out: 'Reactivation of a long-term memory returns the memory to a fragile and labile state, initiating a re-stabilisation process called *reconsolidation*, which allows for updating of the memory.' A client can go back in their mind and 're-vision' an experience, this time from the perspective of their more self-assured adult self.

Working with a therapist with whom they have developed a professional relationship of trust, these new inputs can alter the stored (original) memory, and the 'new' memory can then be *consolidated*. Survival needs—to feel safe, secure and supported—which were unmet at the time of the traumatic experience can now be met and incorporated into the memory. For example, when an adult abuses a child, that child experiences their trauma in the context of a power imbalance so great that they feel there is nothing they can do to change the situation. However, if they revisit the memory as an adult, the balance of power is immediately shifted in the client's favour. They can take more control, re-vision and 'reprogram' the whole experience from a more empowered position, especially when supported and guided by a qualified therapist. As this process progresses, revisiting the traumatic experience gradually becomes less painful, less intimidating and less overwhelming: 'Maladaptive emotions need to be accessed in order to be transformed, in a process that exposes them to new experience and thereby creates new meaning' (Harte, 2019, p. 74). Secondary, maladaptive emotions are bypassed in order to get to the primary emotions associated with survival needs that were not met at the time of the experience. Lingering maladaptive emotional responses that have affected the person negatively every day in conscious and unconscious ways, cease to have the same negative impact on everyday life.

Figure 8: The broadening effect in emotion-focused therapy (EFT)

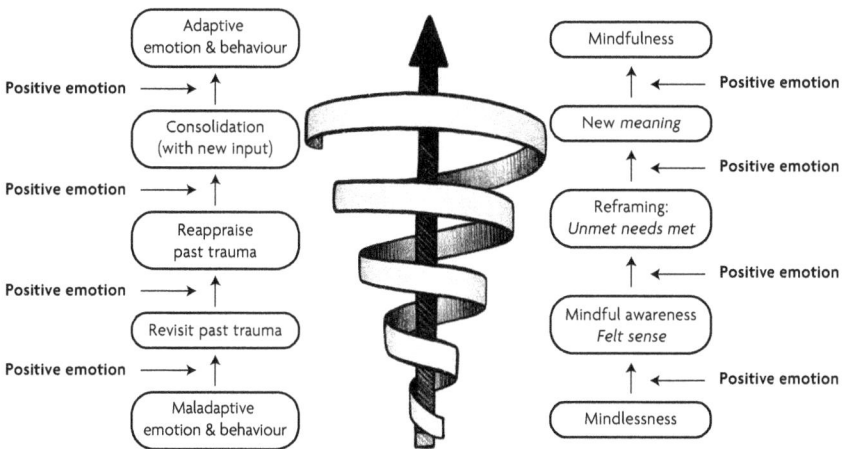

Arntz et al. (2017) promote the idea of *imagery rescripting* as a clinical intervention for painful/traumatic memories, and this has become accepted in mainstream Cognitive Behaviour Therapy. Imagery rescripting has some similarities with EFT in that the basic idea is also to activate memories of emotional trauma. For example, while a therapist guides the process, a client may introduce their adult self into an emotional trauma experienced in childhood and reimagine a different ending. *The adult client is empowered to rewrite the story of events and their associated memories, so that core emotional needs are met, rather than neglected. A change to the meaning of an emotionally traumatic memory is created, without changing the facts of the original trauma.*

In his book *Man's Search for Meaning*, psychiatrist Viktor Frankl explained that finding purpose and meaning in pain can alleviate suffering. Frankl spoke from experience, having been imprisoned and tortured in Nazi concentration camps during the Holocaust. He observed that some people in the camp gave up on life while others pushed through their struggles. Those who gave up, Frankl said, were those who had concluded that there was no point or meaning to life or their suffering, while those who endured were the people who found an answer to the question *Why?* Frankl talks of a 'mass neurotic triad' of aggression, depression, and addiction that occurs when individuals experience an existential vacuum. This vacuum leads to violations of social norms, symptoms of stress, and addiction. Out of his own experience Frankl concluded: *If there is a meaning in life at all, then there must be a meaning in suffering.* Suffering is an ineradicable part of life, as are the tangled threads of fate, and death.

Through meditation practice and due to the neuroplasticity of the brain, neural pathways that were originally laid down as maladaptive responses to past trauma can be altered, and more adaptive responses can be learned.

Case study: EFT and FET combined—Arthur's story

In the following story, emotion-focused therapy and flower essence therapy both played a part in fostering positive changes in neural pathways, which were reflected in a change in emotional state and behaviour, and the capacity to give new *meaning* to past events.

As an example of how memories of past painful experiences can emerge naturally as part of a consultation, I will describe my interaction with a 49-year-old client we will call Arthur. He had consulted with me a number of times over the years, and we had developed a therapeutic relationship of trust. I had grown to understand him and some aspects of his past. During one consultation, in the middle of discussing the possibility and appropriateness of three particular flower essences— Golden Ear Drops, Sunflower and Dogwood—he spontaneously recalled a specific, extremely traumatic experience. He was suddenly 'there' as if it was happening totally in the moment because he was re-experiencing exactly how it *felt*.

As stated already, EFT works with narrative content plus the painful emotions associated with the story. As a therapist, I attend to the interaction between these two so as to decide how best to proceed. Accordingly, as Arthur told his story, at various times I suggested that he take time out so as not to become overwhelmed by the intensity of what he was experiencing. So, between pauses to breathe and self-regulate his painful emotions, he described the following incident that occurred while he was at high school.

Arthur had got into trouble one day and was kept back after class. His father arrived to pick him up, angry and put out about having to be there, and when he walked into the hall and found Arthur chatting with two other classmates who were also on detention for the same incident, he became enraged: 'My dad belted the absolute shit out of me in front of other kids in the hall—no questions asked, nothing said by him as he hit me many times!'

Arthur cried openly when describing this moment, and to allow him to integrate his re-experience of trauma, I suggested time out in what is referred to in EFT as his mental *safe space* (Harte, 2019). Arthur had become a regular meditator, so his safe space occurred in meditation, where he was able to regain his composure and continue. 'My dad didn't even know the full story behind why I was held back at school—he wasn't interested. Later at home he wouldn't let me explain that I had simply been in the wrong place at the wrong time. My dad and mum both gave me the silent treatment all that night and into the next day.'

Arthur revisited his feeling of being totally alone in his terror, humiliation and sense of powerlessness at the hands of his father. None of what he needed at that moment was available—to feel safe and secure, to feel heard and supported, and not to feel humiliated but rather validated. Now, reappraising the experience in the safe environment of the consultation, he had an opportunity to revision and *reframe* it from a more confident and empowered position as an older and wiser adult.

I suggested using two-chair dialogue work, a technique commonly used in EFT. I won't repeat the language used by the now empowered Arthur in his dialogue with his father other than to say he took back a lot of what was taken from him during that childhood experience. Safe and supported in this process, he now felt that some of his primary emotional needs had been acknowledged and met.

Over the next few months of counselling and flower essence therapy—mainly Sunflower and Dogwood (see below)—Arthur came to some level of acceptance, and felt less anger about a number of incidents involving his father, including a family tragedy during which his basic emotional needs had remained unmet. At the age of 9, Arthur's younger sister was hit by a car while playing on the street outside their home, and tragically died as a result. Arthur's parents' way of dealing with this was to immediately send him and his brother off to stay with relatives, without any discussion or attempt to understand how the brothers might be feeling. The boys didn't even attend their sister's funeral, and after returning home, her death was never openly discussed. Once again, emotional support, understanding, and a sense of being heard and validated was not forthcoming.

Fortunately, with the help of EFT and FET, over time, many of Arthur's unmet primary emotional needs resulting from childhood experiences were able to be *felt* and reappraised by him. He learned to integrate his adult self into the re-imagined and reframed experiences— *adult Arthur was empowered to re-write his remembered story of events, so that this time round, his core emotional needs were met, rather than neglected. A change to the meaning of emotionally traumatic memories was createtd, without a change to the facts of the original trauma.* This process was supported by the following three flower essences.

Flower essence for healthy Self-assertion: Sunflower (FES group)

Sunflower flower essence helps to develop healthy assertiveness so that you can *be yourself and stand up for yourself*. It helps bring *confidence* to those who are self-effacing and fearful of displaying their *true worth*, enabling them to '*show some spine*' like the outstanding sunflower plant. It helps both men and women to develop their *positive masculine qualities*.

Negative state
Poor relationship to authority and/or father
Compensatory self-inflation, or self-effacement (FES)

Positive state
Aligned with your inner (higher) authority
Upstanding, honourable and 'your own person'
(Wells, *Essential Flower Essence Book* pp. 330–31)

Flower essence for painful memories: Golden Ear Drops (FES group)

Painful feelings resulting from old hurts, especially the negative emotional charge associated with certain *childhood experiences*, can become entrenched deep in our psyche. Golden Ear Drops flower essence can help us gain a wiser and more comfortable perspective on these *old, painful memories*, allowing us to gain *resolution*. Remember, flower essences help to reveal only what we are prepared, ready and able to understand and accept— our free will always stays intact.

Negative state
Repressed painful memories from childhood
The past undermines current experiences

Positive state
'Releasing painful memories from the past' (FES)
Empowered by one's childhood experience
(Wells, *Essential Flower Essence Book* pp. 191–92)

Flower essence for resilience: Dogwood (FES group)

Dogwood flower essence can help soften a person who has become *scarred and hardened* by unresolved emotional trauma/hurt. Dogwood flower essence helps one become *liberated* from *past emotional injury* and *'freed up'* on emotional, etheric and physical levels.

Negative state
'Scarred' physical/etheric body (psychosomatic conditions)
'Awkward' (FES); 'uncomfortable in your body'

Positive state
'Grace-filled movement' (FES) and coordination
Emotional and physical resilience/flexibility
(Wells, *Essential Flower Essence Book* pp. 169–70)

Humour as therapy

In a therapeutic context, humour is a natural human resource that remains largely untapped, even though humour's psychotherapeutic use is supported by many studies that report its beneficial effect on physical and psychological wellbeing. Laughter and *humour* are now recognised as being therapeutic for many problems. We've all felt better after a good belly laugh. Clowns in hospitals, laughing workshops and humour therapy can have profoundly positive effects on our emotions and on health and wellbeing, especially through their effects on the immune system (Wells, *Essential Flower Essence Book* p. 115).

Figure 9: The broadening effect of humour

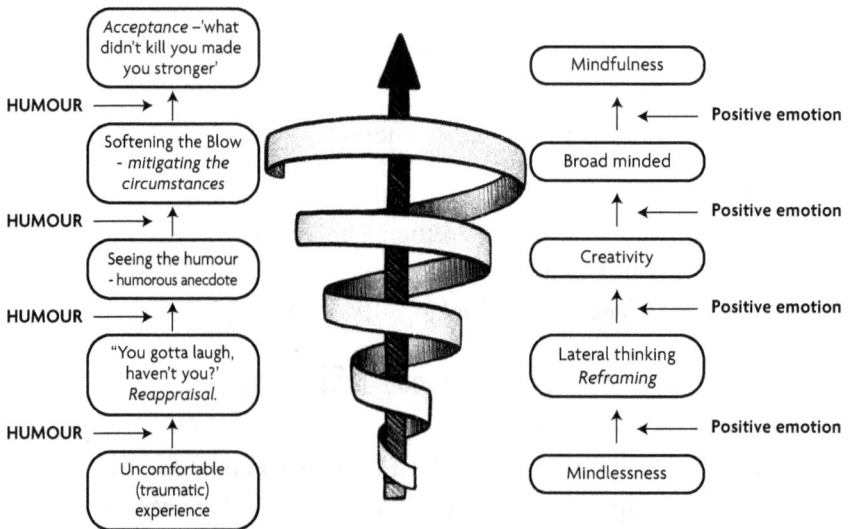

Humour and laughter can increase our experience of positive emotions such as joy, excitement, and happiness, undoing the maladaptive effects of negative emotions and helping us to cope and/or recover better from difficult and traumatic experiences. Laughter releases endorphins and lowers cortisol levels, so that mind and body more easily relax, regardless of circumstances, and mood is elevated. I will share with you two personal experiences in which humour had a significantly therapeutic effect on me, helping me to cope, creatively adapt and recover better from trauma. (I like to think that I do naturally have a good sense of humour—sometimes it works for me and sometimes it gets me into trouble!)

Case study: Heart surgery

When I was around 8 years old, doctors noticed that I had a slightly faulty aortic valve, and suggested that later in life I would most likely need a valve replacement. Fast forward to age 51, when, towards the end of a night of competitive tennis and halfway through my service game, which had been extended because of a number of 'deuces' (40 all), I began to feel very faint. I excused myself and wandered off to the back of the court, sat down, then lay down and promptly lost consciousness—my aortic valve was 85% closed and this had dramatically decreased blood flow to my brain! During the few minutes while I lay unconscious, I had an experience—a vision—that I will try to describe. From my position flat on my back I felt I was looking up (with eyes wide shut!) and saw, hovering in a circle above me, beings who looked down at me with what seemed to be broadly smiling, happy faces—although when I say 'beings' and 'faces,' I'm using human terms to describe ineffable presences who were completely unfamiliar to me but whose joy and warmth I could truly feel. White light spread evenly around them, incredibly bright but warm and calming at the same time. (It was actually a chilly evening—this happened in the middle of winter.) A few of the beings moved their heads in a way that conveyed the message, 'No, not now,' and I knew that this wasn't my time to die.

I know this story will sound farfetched to many, and I can't explain it rationally to myself, but what I felt was vividly clear. I had a profound sense that these presences from the other side found me funny and regarded me with great good humour. While I was unconscious, I had an undeniable experience of powerfully positive emotion, and this sense of euphoria stayed with me after I regained consciousness. This was despite my awareness that my symptoms meant that I would almost certainly now need open heart surgery—very scary, especially at a time when I was living as a single parent with two teenagers at home who relied on me. Nevertheless, I felt buoyed by the experience.

I regained consciousness to the sound of the ambulance siren. The paramedics went about their work conscientiously and considerately, and one of them began to question me to check my state of awareness. Her serious demeanour was in sharp contrast to the cheerful, playful, and mischievous mood I was in, and I had to try my hardest to refrain from making 'dad' jokes and having fun! But, alas, in response to her final question, 'Ok Mark, what is your date of birth?' I couldn't help myself and replied, fully of aware of what I was saying, '17th of the 11th, 1855,' which would have made me over 150 years old! She looked at me in disbelief, and when I said, 'Nahhh, just kidding,' she smiled too.

I know there are those who interpret near-death experiences like mine as the hallucinations of an oxygen-starved brain—in my case due to aortic stenosis. What this interpretation does not take into account is the life-changing effect of the very real FELT experience. Indisputably, the sense of joy, warmth and humour communicated to me while I was unconscious enabled me to maintain a positive take on what was transpiring, so that I coped better with a serious and potentially disablingly traumatic experience.

Case study: Vasectomy!

A second experience (not as profound as the first!) relates to when I had a vasectomy. Once again a sense of humour kept me buoyed with positive emotion during an anxiety-producing, potentially traumatic time. I arrived at a small private hospital a little earlier than expected on the morning of my procedure and was directed to a room where I undressed, put on the hospital gown they gave me and hopped into bed. Around 30 mins later I heard the doctor who was to do the surgery arrive at reception. Unaware that I was already present and within earshot, he said to the nurse, 'I wonder where my patient is—I'm operating on some naturopathic character today.' Hearing this, I felt sudden apprehension in the groin area! With adrenalin egging me on, I called out, 'He's already here!' There was a long pause, then the nurse replied, 'Good, thank you Mr Wells.' I thought, 'Uh-oh, we're off to a great start.' It was quite a while before he came to my room for a rather awkward pre-op briefing. Fast forward and I'm on the operating table with a curtain preventing me from seeing any of the surgical 'goings on' down below—I had chosen to have a local, rather than the full anaesthetic the doctor had recommended, and which in hindsight, probably would have been better.

When the doctor began operating, all I could see was the assisting nurse and himself, from the waist up. Moments later, I became aware that he was pointing what seemed to me, in my anxious state, to be an oversized syringe at my private parts—or not so private at this point—and saying, 'OK Mark, just a little prick!' Once again, humour came to my emotional rescue and, pretending to take his statement as an appraisal, I said, 'Ohhh, thanks very much!' I'm not sure if he got the joke but the nurse definitely had a smirk on her face. Seeing the humorous side of the situation distracted me and helped me feel more relaxed from that point on through an operation that was at times very uncomfortable for various reasons. I believe that once again, negative impacts were *mitigated* by humour, which ultimately helped me to make a quicker recovery. The other definite upside was that I had a good story to tell at the dinner table! But now if anyone asks, I tell them if they're having a vasectomy they should go for a full anaesthetic.

Flower essence for buoyant courage: Borage (FES group)

Here's an essence that shows the broadening effect of FET and (good) humour combined. Borage flower essence can help one regain or develop a better sense of humour, or at least become more good-humoured. Borage has been valued throughout history for its ability to promote cheerfulness and courage and can be a catalyst in the process of lightening up and learning to look on the bright side of life.

Negative state
Succumbing to the pessimistic ('glass half empty') view
Becoming discouraged/resigned when facing personal challenges

Positive state
'When the going gets tough, the tough get going!'
'Buoyant courage and optimism' (FES)
Positivity in the face of personal challenge
(Wells, *Essential Flower Essence Book* p. 114)

Case study: Pets

The following true story is a sad one but it has a humorous and thought-provoking angle—it shows how animals don't know that flower essences aren't meant to work! Flower essences are helpful to animals as well as humans, and Borage can help people—and their pets—display resilience in the darkest moments, as the following story shows. I recall a situation in which I prescribed Borage flower essence for a grief-stricken young dog. Two puppies, Ben and Bobby, were bought by widowed twin sisters Mary and Patricia when they retired and moved from Sydney to live in country Victoria. The puppies were brothers from the same litter, and immediately became a much-loved part of the family. Then tragedy struck! Both dogs escaped over the front fence and one of the brothers, Ben, ran onto a busy highway and was struck by a car and killed. Of course Mary and Patricia were extremely upset, but the surviving dog, Bobby, was inconsolable, moping around the back yard with his head drooping, not eating, and obviously deep in mourning. Mary asked me whether there was something natural that she could give him to ease some of his pain. I suggested Borage flower essence, and told her to give it to Bobby every 15–30 minutes for the rest of the day and get back to me tomorrow to reassess. But Mary rang me back that same afternoon and told me, 'After three doses, Bobby's demeanour changed dramatically, and although he's not fully back to his playful self, he is engaging with me and Patricia more and has started eating again. I don't know how, but he has even lifted our spirits! Can we take some of the drops too?'

Here I want to stress once more that flower essences don't suppress or bury feelings, they allow us to call on resources and abilities we already have within us. A new positivity creates a *broadening effect* that enables these strengths to come to the fore to help us adapt, cope better and display *'buoyant courage and optimism'* (FES) and *positivity in the face of personal challenge*. Positive emotions did not replace, remove or suppress the grief felt by Bobby (or Mary and Patricia), but it did change the emotional balance, so that grief no longer overwhelmed and incapacitated them.

The importance of the therapeutic relationship

Throughout this book I've mentioned the vital need for establishing a relationship of trust between therapist and client, and at this point I want to emphasise its importance once more. I have described therapeutic 'tools' in the form of EFT, meditation and FET that people can use to help heal the effects of painful emotional experiences in the past, and successfully navigate current and future experiences of suffering. However, raising awareness, processing, working through, and healing major emotional trauma will always be more effective, and most importantly safer, when carried out within the bond of trust created in a good therapeutic relationship with an appropriately qualified therapist. Arousing deeply felt emotions related to past trauma requires empathetic understanding, skilful guidance and management and a strong *therapeutic presence* that can help clients to identify, explore, make sense of, transform and flexibly manage their emotions (Greenberg et al., 2007). During and after a therapeutic session, flower essence and meditation therapies can be used to enhance and consolidate the ongoing process.

> *Therapeutic presence* is a way of *being* that optimises the doing and techniques of therapy. TP provides clients with a sense of safety, allowing them to be seen, heard, understood, and 'feel felt,' while also strengthening the therapeutic alliance. TP invites therapists to work on their own balance of presence and compassion with self and clients, ensuring they remain centred and effective even in the face of difficult emotions. This type of relationship helps regulate clients' emotions and supports their movement towards emotional health and neurophysiological integration. (Shari Geller, 2024)

HARNESSING EMOTION TO CREATE YOUR DESIRED REALITY
4th dimension of EI: Using emotions to facilitate performance

The fourth dimension of EI relates to the ability to make use of emotions adaptively by directing them toward constructive activities and personal performance. A person who is highly capable in this respect is able to:

- *self-motivate* to continuously do better, by allowing emotions to inform them about their needs, values, goals and life purpose
- use emotions to help manage difficult circumstances and *cope in positive and productive ways*
- use emotions to help *influence and manage social relationships*

Emotionally intelligent people know how to use their emotions to support a successful, purposeful life that is in line with their values so that they can reach their goals and grow personally.

Using emotion to Self-motivate

Emotions can enhance performance through providing self-motivation. The experience of an emotion can motivate an individual to take a certain course of action: anger, for instance, may motivate a person to push back against a transgressor, while the experience of joy may motivate a person to continue engaging in a certain activity. Emotions move and motivate us (Lang and Bradley, 2010) and in fact the words emotion, move, and motivate share the same Latin root—*emovare*, meaning 'to move.' In general, positive emotions such as pride or joy motivate us to *approach* or *seek out* the experience we think has triggered the emotion. For instance, when we feel enjoyment and enthusiasm during a tennis game (emotional trigger), we may become very motivated to continue playing this game—we *approach* or *seek it out*. However, when we experience emotions such as anger and contempt, they typically motivate us to respond to their trigger by *opposing* or *avoiding* it. For instance, when a person says something that offends us (emotional trigger), our anger may motivate us to insult (oppose) that person or walk away from (avoid) them or both. When we feel shame and embarrassment after being ridiculed by a colleague (emotional trigger) this may trigger social withdrawal (avoidance), and motivate us to stay away from them in the future. And then there are emotions such as sadness that often do not motivate either approach or avoidance of the emotional trigger, but rather result in *inactivity*. For instance, the sadness and rejection felt after a relationship breakup (emotional trigger) may result in *passivity* or *being unreceptive* to the possibility of new relationships—although a period of inaction may be best, to allow time to contemplate and reassess rather than jumping in again too soon!

Impulsive responses

People may be motivated to *approach*, *avoid*, or *withdraw* from experiences they believe have triggered emotions—action tendencies that are driven by the emotions that are felt. Here, emotion dictates an impulsive course of *reaction* rather than a conscious choice, and when these emotion-driven behaviours become habitual, they can have the paradoxical effect of keeping maladaptive emotions alive or even exacerbating them. For instance, when people who fear rejection succumb to their fear and avoid socialising, it creates social isolation—the exact situation they initially feared. Research has shown that aggression intensifies anger (McKay et al., 2003), avoidance can create anxiety disorders (Allen et al., 2008), and withdrawal is the prime driver of depression (Zettel, 2007). This negative spiral is another example of 'What you resist will persist!'

It is important for people to learn that acting on the impulse that accompanies an emotion strengthens the emotion by giving it 'free rein,' empowering it to take over. Emotion-driven behaviour, regardless of how right or natural it feels, is usually counterproductive. The ideal way to respond is mindfully, not mindlessly in an impulsive way, and make better choices in your behavioural response to emotions. I have mentioned often how a major flow-on from regular practice of meditation is a more mindful approach to everyday life. Here are some examples of specific flower essences that can help us become more mindful and hence make better decisions rather than impulsive ones, by fostering a positive, ultimately more adaptive, change in perspective.

Flower essence for harmonious responsiveness: Tiger Lily (FES group)

Anger can lead to aggression and confrontation, which can lead to more anger. Tiger Lily flower essence can help to break that cycle.

Negative state
'Overly aggressive; excessive yang forces' (FES)
Power struggles; 'separatist tendencies' (FES

Positive state
Capacity for cooperation—enhanced feminine/receptive energy (FES)
Win/win mentality—living in harmony
(Wells, *Essential Flower Essence Book* p. 340)

Flower essence for renewed interest in life: Wild Rose (Bach group)

Wild Rose can disrupt the cycle of depression, withdrawal, and inactivity, that leads to feelings of greater depression.

Negative state
Withdrawn resignation
Disinterested and dispirited

Positive state
Enthusiastic and involved
Renewed interest and passion for life
(Wells, *Essential Flower Essence Book* p. 367)

Flower essence for facing our fears: Mimulus (Bach group)

Mimulus flower essence can help to break the cycle in which fear leads to avoidance and isolation, which leads to more fear.

Negative state
Mental fears
Dread of everyday things

Positive state
Quiet courage and strength
Acceptance of life's inherent risks
(Wells, *Essential Flower Essence Book* p. 241)

People stuck in maladaptive, emotion-driven behaviours can also benefit from a technique used in Dialectical Behaviour Therapy called 'Opposite to Emotion' or 'Opposite Action' that helps them get unstuck. This technique directs clients to act in ways that are opposite to the behaviours toward which their difficult emotions drive them, generally bringing quick relief. For example, a client who feels guilty because they did something hurtful to another person may initially try to hide from this person or avoid accepting responsibility for their actions. Using 'Opposite to Emotion' encourages this person to mindfully *approach rather than avoid* the other person. They can then apologise and attempt to make the situation better. Another example of engaging in 'Opposite Action' is when fear is driving you towards retreat or avoiding a situation.

Case study: Opposite action to overcome fear of public speaking

As mentioned earlier, when I was young I had an intense fear of public speaking and for many years managed to avoid it at any cost. Eventually, however, that cost became too high! The emotional frustration of not fulfilling my deeply felt desire to become a health practitioner, to help people and be of service to society, became more intense than my anxiety about speaking in public. I had become *motivated to oppose my fear-driven avoidance*. Emotions of longing that arose from a deep level revealed that in the *now*, my *values and sense of purpose* had become *more important motivators for my behaviour than my past need to stay hidden*—and I was able to use Garlic flower essence to support me in moving in the opposite direction from where my fear had driven me.

An emotional response doesn't emerge unless there is something important—something of *value*—for the individual to be aware of. In other words, emotions reveal information about our values—the things we consider to be important, such as accountability, achievement, altruism, ambition, creativity, enthusiasm, equality, exploration, and autonomy. By the time I was ready to confront my fear of public speaking, I had come to cherish many of these values, which related to my desire to find purpose through being of service to the world as a health practitioner. Using this example from my life we can see how it is possible to use awareness of emotion to bring about adaptive change:

- Firstly, I became aware of the feedback loop in which the more I stayed stuck in old patterns and avoided the challenge of public speaking, the more fearful I became.

- Secondly, with time I became aware of emotions that were deeper and stronger than my fear, connected to my desire to express my values and find a sense of purpose.

Emotions therefore can be understood as *data* and when interpreted correctly can, amongst other things, inform us about how closely our life is aligning with our deep personal *needs, values* and, in my case, *sense of purpose*. Negative emotions such as shame, regret or guilt can inform us that our actions are incongruent with our *values* (see Mullein below). The ability to extract this information allows us to use emotions as signals and motivating forces in the service of our development.

Flower essence for openness to inner guidance: Mullein (FES group)

Mullein people are unsure about who they are and are easily defined by others' expectations, especially peers. They are indecisive when making choices for themselves as they can't seem to connect with their inner guidance or morality (FES). If we use our feelings/emotions as *signals that are in the service of our values and goals*, their guidance will help us grow, express our true self, and thereby display our unique and full potential.

Negative state
'Inability to hear one's inner voice' (FES)—confused
In denial of one's truth

Positive state
Integrity—receptive to inner guidance and *emotional signals*
Uprightness through alignment with one's *values and goals*

Using emotions to help manage difficult circumstances

Emotions can enhance performance and facilitate goal achievement if we understand the function and consequences of positive and negative feeling states. We have described how the function of positive emotions differs fundamentally from the function of negative emotions. Just as negative emotions cause a narrowing of thoughts to focus on the specifics of a problem, positive emotions expand thought-action repertoires and lateral thinking capacity. Also, we have seen how positive emotions encourage an upward spiral of further positivity according to Fredrickson's Broaden and Build theory. Generating positive emotions directly promotes goal achievement by enhancing our creative responses to life situations. Positive emotions enable people to generate creative solutions to goal-related challenges, encouraging them to think laterally and consider alternative pathways towards their goals. For example, as described earlier, Pansy flower essence can remind someone who has been unwell for some time how to think outside the mental inhibitions of an illness so as to be more open to the possibility of feeling fully well again. Pansies have traditionally been given to cheer someone up after having faced a personal challenge. The person receiving pansies would feel a sense of joy and optimism. This is not a false hope for a sudden or complete recovery but an opening and elevation of the mind to a different perspective on health and wellbeing (Wells, *Essential Flower Essence Book* p. 267).

When we make a creative choice and decide to take a certain path, emotions play a critical role in helping us commit to the choices/decisions we make. Much research has gone into how to make the best decisions but, in the end, what is most important is to *make the best of your decisions*, i.e. make the decisions right. In addition to helping us make decisions, emotions play a critical role in helping us commit to the choices we make. To move forward with a decision, we need what Professor Baba Shiv calls *decision confidence*—the conviction that our choice is the correct one.

Throughout his career, Baba Shiv, Professor of Marketing at Stanford Graduate School of Business, has researched how brain structures related to emotion and motivation affect the choices we make. In a 2024 interview conducted at the Stanford Graduate School of Business, Shiv explains that the rational brain is only responsible for about 5–10% of our decision-making, whereas emotions are about 90% responsible. 'Emotions ... have a profound influence on our decisions and we aren't aware of it,' he states. Much of society, especially business, places a premium on rational thinking, but Shiv encourages us to embrace our instincts and intuitions. He concludes that when it comes to decision-making, it is much better to think like an artist. 'If you emerge from the decision with doubts, you're more likely to give up too early and not persist in the course of action that you adopted,' Shiv says. 'You need to emerge from the decision FEELING absolutely confident. It's not making the "right decision" but making the decision right.' Generating positive emotions can help one *cope* with doubts or setbacks on the road to one's goal. Resilient people better understand the benefits of positive emotions and *harness* these benefits to their advantage to effectively cope with negative emotional experiences.

Harnessing humour, FET, and meditation

Humour is one of my personal favourites among emotions that can be productively harnessed, because of the way it can elicit further positive emotions to help regulate negatively emotional situations. Spending time with a friend who makes you laugh or simply seeing the humour in your own difficult experiences can elicit positive emotions that help you cope better, as described earlier. In the same way, meditation and/or FET can enable you to feel better by offering a more positive and mindful perspective. Remaining optimistic (hopeful rather than hopeless!) ensures resilience after setbacks. Regular meditation practice ensures that you develop a more mindful perspective, and this *broad-minded* approach to life allows you to understand, gain perspective and come to a better *acceptance* of your challenges, and so cope better and display resilience.

Flower essence for resilience after setbacks: Gentian (Bach group)

Gentian flower essence helps when we have become discouraged and disheartened by setbacks in achieving our hopes and aspirations, particularly when we have worked hard for them. It helps people to remain optimistic and hopeful, enabling a broad perspective on the setbacks they have experienced. For instance, you could view your progress in a wider timeline and see that even though you have come up short this time, you came much closer than in your previous attempt. Is your glass half full or half empty?

Negative state
Depressed; narrow-minded view of problems
Discouraged by setbacks

Positive state
Ability to oversee and understand—broad-minded perspective
Resilient—undeterred by setbacks
(Wells, *Essential Flower Essence Book* p. 189)

Using emotions to influence/manage social relationships

Emotions can enhance performance if we understand how our expression of emotions influences the emotions of others. Most people have experienced a situation in which their own expression of an emotion caused another person to experience the *same* emotion, and vice-versa: emotions can be contagious (Dimitroff et al., 2017). Our emotions can also induce *different* emotions in others: when one person expresses anger, another who witnesses it may feel fear; an expression of gratitude may evoke feelings of pride in the receiver. Emotionally intelligent people can use their emotional awareness to influence their social environment and so move towards personal and group goals.

Flower essence for motivating others: Larkspur (FES group)

Larkspur enables you to foster contagious enthusiasm, and act with a greater feeling of generosity, altruism and 'an inner joyfulness which energises others' (FES). Whether in the family, at work or in a community group, everyone learns to accept responsibility, inspired and motivated by your natural leadership qualities and charisma.

Negative state
Inflated sense of self-importance
Overburdened by sense of duty and obligation; may become resentful

Positive state
Altruistic, *'charismatic leadership'* (FES)
Enthusiastic, generous, 'joyful service' (FES)
(Wells, *Essential Flower Essence Book* p. 225)

In summary, positive emotions facilitate progress toward goals by enhancing the ability to cope with setbacks or roadblocks. Emotionally intelligent people use the feedback from their emotional responses to know firstly whether they are heading in the right direction, and secondly how they can use their emotions to support this progress. They re-think and adjust their course of action when negative emotions are experienced, and use positive emotions to increase their *decision confidence* and commit to their creative choices. Later in the book, I describe how I adjusted my course of action when faced with the need for a heart valve replacement by being proactive in researching all my options. If I had resigned myself to accepting a mechanical valve as initially suggested by my heart specialist, I would have found it very difficult to lift myself out of my own negative emotional response. So instead of resigning myself, I decided to investigate all possibilities and began an intensive internet search. The hope of finding a way forward—one that satisfied my need, and was aligned with my values and life purpose—generated such positive emotion in me that I was able to overcome my fears, re-evaluate my situation and commit whole*heart*edly (excuse the pun!) to my research. And after hours of browsing, I found the information I had been looking for—a heart-valve replacement option called the Ross Procedure, which absolutely suited my needs.

Synergy between EI dimensions

Although the different skills that are essential for EI have been described separately, in reality, they work together synergistically. No-one can express emotions if they are not aware of feeling them in the first place. And, one must be able to emotionally self-regulate in order to harness emotions to facilitate goal achievement. If emotions such as anger and frustration overwhelm us in pursuit of our goals, how can we keep going? We must self-regulate. Also, EI skills are interlinked, and improving one EI skill will positively enhance another.

My 5th dimension of EI: Harnessing emotion to create your desired life

Emotion is the creative and transformative force in life. As psychotherapist Mihaela Ivan Holtz puts it: 'You need to access your emotions to make your art, perform, or accomplish your goals. Emotions are your creative power' (Creative Minds). The writer Arnold Bennett goes further, stating: 'There can be no knowledge without emotion. ... To the cognition of the brain must be added the experience of the soul' (*Journals*, 1932). The quality of our consciousness in any given moment determines who we are now and in the future. Wise thinkers throughout the ages have suggested that the substance of the world and the essential dynamic of time is imbued with a *purposeful force*, often understood as a divine impulse that drives the cycles and rounds of evolution. On a microcosmic level, an individual's time is also infused with this *tension of transformation*, and we can avail ourselves of it more fully if we make a conscious choice to do so. Naturopathy and other forms of natural healing understand that we are made aware of this tension and impulse towards transformation through our disease symptoms. When we follow Nature Cure practices and principles, we tap into the inherent self-organising and healing processes of all living systems, to enable physical, emotional and mental *transformation* towards better health and wellbeing. Humanistic psychology recognises this tension of transformation when it emphasises that individuals possess an inherent drive towards self-actualisation and creativity.

Carl Rogers and Abraham Maslow, titans in the humanistic movement, believed that human beings are born with the desire to grow, create and love, and possess the power to direct their own lives. Carl Jung saw this intrinsic transformational force in the individual's process of self-realisation, and their discovery and experience of meaning and purpose; this force is the means by which one finds oneself and becomes who one really is, and has always desired to be. The process of *individuation*, as Jung refers to it, is never-ending. Far from being selfish, an individuated person feels deeper responsibility to support and serve others, to foster peace, and grow (*transform*) to wholeness and integrity. Here, at a microcosmic, individual level, we 'come back around' and re-align more consciously with the tension of transformation, so that we are driven and nourished by it at a macrocosmic level.

Giving thought to what is possible focuses the human will (power) in the present to bring about transformation in the future. Focused imaginative thought, fortified repeatedly by the *creative force of emotion* and our deepest desire, adds *the experience of the soul* to *the cognition of the brain*. This allows us to catch and ride the wave of transformation that radiates through all the structures and systems of relationship in the world, to create our desired life. Ken Wilber's book *No boundary: Eastern and Western approaches to personal growth* (2001) expresses this understanding that there are no boundaries in the universe. Boundaries are illusions, products of the way we try to map and edit our reality. They may help us to get a sense of our own territory, but reality is not so confined. All boundaries and personal territories are *permeable*, and so the *tension of transformation* flows throughout (us) all.

'If you change the way you look at things, the things you look at change' (Max Planck). We can't directly control our external environment, but we can control some aspects of our internal one, which, ironically, then controls how we creatively view and influence our external environment. To change the way we look at things outside ourselves, we need to change the way we look at things within. 'Who looks outside, dreams; who looks inside, awakes' (Carl Jung). If you change your focus and look within yourself, you will change what you become. 'Where focus goes, energy flows. And where energy flows, whatever you're focusing on grows' (Tony Robbins). Wherever you focus attention, that's where you are devoting time, energy, and feeling, and that is what nourishes and shapes growth. Where you place your attention becomes your reality! Moving your focus away from what is outside you and out of your control, to what is inside you and in your control, you concentrate your attention on the goals and values, the strengths and weaknesses, the feelings and desires that make you the person you are. Without this self-awareness we become distracted from what we are truly passionate about and what provides meaning for us, and become more susceptible to pressures externally applied by society, our family and our friends and peers.

You increase your freedom to change how you look at things if you approach them *mindfully* in the present moment. However, you will never be fully present if your existence is disturbed or encroached upon by the past, whether consciously or subconsciously. If your mind 'carries a heavy burden of the past' in the form of unresolved emotional pain, your future will remain 'a replica of the past … [which] perpetuates itself through [your] lack of presence' (Tolle, 2018). The quality of your *Self*-consciousness—the concept you have of your *Self*—depends on how unfettered by the past your mind is, in the present. This determines the quality of the present and your future.

As I have described many times throughout this book, FET, meditation and EFT can enable us to be more mindful and grounded in the present moment. Re-viewing, processing and healing past emotionally traumatic experiences through these therapies means we can literally rewire our brain, and change the maladaptive neural pathways generated during these past experiences into ones that are more adaptive. We are freed up to experience a more mindful sense of presence. The past no longer contaminates the present to perpetuate more of the same in the future. We are *free* from our heavy burdens— the 'baggage' of the past—free to create the life we desire *now*.

Creating our future for better or for worse

The concept that we construct our own perceptions of others' emotions (Fieldman Barrett, 2017) and our world in general, implies that we can be the architects of our emotional experiences. Preconception and interoception—how we are informed by our past and present emotional experiences—work together to (instantaneously) create our experience of reality—how it feels right NOW. Psychologists can tell you that it's not necessarily people, events and circumstances but your perception that determines your personal reality. *Our past (traumatic) emotional experiences can contaminate what we feel and experience in the present. This can interfere with our creativity and our ability to accomplish the reality we desire.*

Example: Perception as an influence for the worse

Earlier I told the hypothetical story of someone (later helped with Scarlet Monkeyflower flower essence) who missed his freeway turnoff because he was angry and aggrieved by what he throught another driver had 'done to him' a few minutes earlier. As a result, he arrived late for an important meeting and missed an opportunity. He was distracted from being (mindfully) in the present moment by what had transpired in the past. Past emotional experiences, whether recent or distant, can strongly influence our consciousness for better and for worse.

> A strong unconscious emotional pattern may manifest as an external event that appears to just happen to you. For example, I have observed that people who carry a lot of anger inside without being aware of it and without expressing it are more likely to be attacked, verbally or even physically, by other angry people, and often for no apparent reason. They have a strong emanation of anger that certain people pick up subliminally and that triggers their own latent anger. (Tolle, 2018, p. 21)

I have spoken often in this book about how when we are 'stuck' in maladaptive emotional reactions/behaviours we are limited in our capacity to change our lives for the better. I have also spoken about how by introducing positive (adaptive) emotions into our maladaptive emotional responses through therapies such as FET, meditation or EFT, we can transform maladaptive responses into adaptive ones. We have described how emotions are crucial in motivating behaviour— you more often do what you feel like doing than what reason or logic dictates or what you 'think' you want to do. If you want to make a decision to do something it must *feel* right, so that you have 'decision confidence' for the best results. If you want to achieve change you need to change the emotions that have been motivating you to stay the same. Emotions deeply influence thought. To help people change what they think, therapists must help them change what they feel.

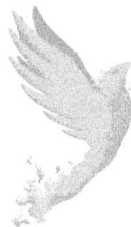

Case study: Perception as an influence for the better

From my early twenties I have had a great desire to build a therapeutic practice in which I could do what I love doing—consulting and helping clients create health and wellbeing. *When students, other practitioners, accountants and marketing experts have asked me over the years, 'How do you attract clients to your practice?' I used to reply, 'Word of mouth.' But to be honest my answer was only half-true. I would now add, 'and by taking Willow flower essence!'* This essence has been a godsend for improving my ability to cope and display resilience. I will describe one of many instances of how it has helped me.

When my children were 14 and 15 and living with me as a single parent, I self-prescribed Willow to help shift a mood that had begun to consume me! I was working with my clients from home, my teenagers were being teenagers, time for myself was non-existent. Further, when I looked ahead I saw only a few client appointments booked, and I had some big bills coming up! I was emotionally drained, irritable, worried and feeling like a victim: 'Poor me! Why do I have to do everything?'

My negative mood was affecting how I related to my kids because my tolerance was at an all-time low. And I must have also been sending this mood out 'through the ether' to potential clients because they stayed away! Fortunately, I said to myself, 'Hang on! I need to practice what I preach if I want to change things for the better!' So I took stock of my life and did what I needed to do to enable me to bounce back. The first step was taking Willow flower essence. Within 24 hours my attitude had become more positive and I felt a noticeable lift in my mood. Then what was happening around me began to change. The dynamic between me and my kids improved and our responses to one another became much more civil. I was no longer irritable, and became far less reactive. I had regained my self-belief and *felt* much more positive about my family life and my practice, with a clearer picture of what was needed. And with that the phone began to ring as clients contacted me to make appointments. Not only my kids but my clients, on some level, were responding positively to the fact that what I was 'giving off' had improved! Willow enabled me to transform my mood into something more positive at a deep, subconscious level. This change within me, although subtle, resulted in significant changes in my outer life, in the form of better relationships and an upturn in client bookings. I've never figured out how to explain all this to my accountant!

Flower essence for freedom from resentment: Willow (Bach group)

Willow flower essence helps to foster resilience after hurts and setbacks, so that we don't get stuck in resentment and feelings of being a victim. The consequence, especially in my case as described above, is the manifestation of better, more desired life circumstances.

Negative state
Victim mentality—'poor me'
Wallowing in resentment—'why me?'

Positive state
Self-determination
Emotional resilience
(Wells, *Essential Flower Essence Book* p. 369)

Fully feeling your desired reality now

Memories are malleable and constantly undergo revision. However, the degree to which emotional responses become disorganised, maladaptive and resistant to change by subsequent life experiences (and/or therapies) depends on how early they were experienced, how intensely they were felt (how much emotion was evoked—the degree of arousal) and how frequently they and the situations activating them occurred (Greenberg, qtd. in Lane et al., 2015). If the present effect of our past emotional experiences is highly dependent on how intensely emotions were felt and how frequently they occurred, let's use this understanding to create and reinforce the emotional experiences and reality that we want to be our future. If we can imagine and *feel* our desired future frequently and intensely, we lessen our resistance to change. I therefore pose the question: If we can change the experience of our past, *now*, what's to stop us from changing our experience of our future? If we can *re-construct* our past for the better, why can't we *construct* our future for the better?

To feel your desired future, sort out your priorities in life, including your needs, values, passions, and what is meaningful and gives you a sense of purpose. These are the qualities that will arouse and evoke intensely positive emotions in you, which is essential to change the experience of your present and future. To change the intense emotional pain associated with past trauma, we need to evoke a similar intensity of positive emotions if we are to heal and render our painful memories malleable enough to undergo re-evaluation, revision and reconstruction. What is most important to you? Is it your family? Your career? Your service to humanity? All of the above? Let your needs, values and meaningful goals inform you about what you really want, so that you can imagine a desired future that aligns with your truth and not necessarily with the ex*pectations of outside influences.* If you are currently committed to something in your life that did not arise from your own inner desire but primarily satisfies someone else's expectations—for example those of society or of a parent—you are highly unlikely to be able to maintain your commitment. Or, if you do, you will never be fully satisfied with what you achieve. Anthony Chiminello puts it this way: 'When you are not clear on your values or beliefs, then you tend to subordinate to other people's values and outside influences, losing the freedom to be your true self' (Bridgeworld International). It will never feel truly authentic, and you will feel like an imposter—never fulfilled or content until you are living up to the expectations of your true Self.

Visualise how things would look if you were living your desired life, whether as a 'big picture' or in some smaller but significant area. Every time you revisit your vision during the day, let the details come to you and make adjustments if need be. Allow your imagined ideal life to take shape by itself and become more and more vivid in your mind. When you let go of trying to control your vision, you become more open to manifesting *serendipity*. The term serendipity, coined by English novelist Horace Walpole, describes the accidental discovery of something valuable. This phenomenon tends to create unexpected cumulative results from a combination of desire, focus, persistence, mindful broadmindedness and *flexibility*, often while looking for one thing and finding another. The potential of 'accidental' discoveries is heightened when we engage intentionally in the process of designing our most desired life. Merton and Barber (2004) describe it well: 'The observer [comes] to the datum rather than [bringing] the datum to [them].' This describes your journey from a *felt* fantasy to fact.

Practise over and over again exactly how it would *feel* to be where you desire to be in life, even if it is a struggle at first. Over time, you will get a much stronger *felt sense* of what it's like in that desired place. It is essential to make a practice of brief reverie a regular and recurring part of your day, when you *feel*, for a moment, how it is to be in your ideal job, to live in your ideal house, to spend time with your ideal friend, to have resolved your differences with your sister or father etc. It is not enough to just visualise your desired reality, although that is essential— you have to *feel* the emotion of it as *already* being your reality. This creative, *impassioned* use of imagination can make manifest the vision of what you desire. The more often you can conjure and remain with this growing feeling inside yourself, the faster it will come to life outside you. The more strongly you can *feel* it, the closer it is to becoming your reality, consistent with your values and what is deeply meaningful for you. You need to be dedicated to it, but, at the same time, stay open-minded enough to be able to adapt and rejig it ever so slightly when necessary to keep it just right!

Previously I proposed that if the effect of our emotional experiences in the past is highly dependent on how intensely they were felt and how frequently they occurred, this means that we can use this understanding to create and make more permanent the emotional experiences and reality we want to *be* our future. If we can imagine and *feel* intensely, we lessen our resistance to change—whether it be for the better, the same or worse. And further, one doesn't have to have any specific conscious intent. Every time we feel intensely, even just daydreaming about *being* in a certain life situation, good or bad, we are incrementally lessening our resistance to it becoming our reality. It becomes a self-fulfilling prophecy. And further, there may even be an advantage to not having any conscious intent or belief, as this can eliminate the second-guessing and resistance created by an overly rational mind. Meditation and FET used therapeutically can enable you to engage more deeply in this life-changing process and support you when the going gets tough. We all need all the help we can get!

Meditation and creative imagination

Regular practice of meditation can indirectly help you create your desired life. Every time you meditate you get better at *not resisting and just accepting;* you learn not to (over) try, and you get better at allowing yourself to just *be*. So when you daydream or immerse yourself in your ideal vision and/or safe space in your mind on a regular basis, your resistance to it becoming reality wanes over time. The quality of pure consciousness is experienced in those daydreaming moments more easily because in meditation you have often already experienced just *being* without resistance. The vision or dream is uncontaminated by your past or present circumstances, and continually shapes an existence that resembles more and more closely what you desire.

The late Dr Melissa Harte often referred to a simple meditation and mindfulness 'grounding and safe place' technique she developed, observing that 'people who engage in the … technique to regulate their arousal levels on a very regular basis actually improve more quickly than those who do not' (2019 p. 87). The ability to better regulate arousal levels enables people to be 'more present' in the moment, embodying it, and so counteracts any 'habit of disassociation' (p. 87). One of the key aspects of emotional intelligence is the ability to self-regulate one's emotion, and to stay in the present moment to fully feel it, without allowing it to take over or overwhelm us. We can therefore be informed by it and/or harness it to enhance performance in the areas we desire.

In your musings, reflections or daydreams, if you *feel* intensely that you are really *present* in a life that is *better*, *worse* or *similar*, and you experience this often, it inevitably will become your reality. But there's more! If, for whatever reason, you are taking appropriate flower essences and/or regularly meditating, during those reflective times, you will experience more positive and clearer visions of your reality—you will get more of what you desire, coincidently and as a consequence.

Flower essence for groundedness: Blackberry (FES group)

I have found that Blackberry flower essence stands out for its ability to enable people to make what they want happen in their lives. The blackberry plant is very resilient, tenacious and persistent. The flower essence helps us develop persistence, patience and the discipline required to achieve any worthwhile goal. Just as we must wait for the fruit to ripen to full sweetness, we must persist and endure difficulties so that we may ultimately taste the sweetness of victory (Wells, *Essential Flower Essence Book* p. 106).

Negative state
Procrastination—'where do I start?'
'Inability to translate goals and ideals into concrete action' (FES)

Positive state
Purposeful and decisive action
Resilient, tenacious and 'fully grounded'

Changing our reality by harnessing emotion is *not magic*, it happens within us and our lives every day in all sorts of minor and major ways. We are the architects of our emotional experience of life. We construct our own perceptions of our world, and that ultimately determines our reality. We are what we *feel* about our *Self*!

USING POSITIVE EMOTIONS CREATIVELY

The cosmic meaning of consciousness became overwhelmingly clear to me ... that man is indispensable for the completion of the creation; that, in fact, he himself is the second creator of the world. (Carl Jung, qtd. in Dunne, 2015 p. 92)

Case study: Gabby—a new life ...

Gabby had been coming to see me at the practice several times a year for over five years about different health issues. There was a common theme around problems related to her gut; Gabby was a highly sensitive person, and this was reflected in the sensitivity of her digestive system. During consultations, she would often refer in passing to her difficult childhood, but when I offered her space and opportunity to talk more about it she would reply, 'That's in the past, you can't dwell on it' or, 'Another time maybe—I just want to get myself well now.' I never pushed it because, firstly, I respect each individual's right to decide what, if anything, they wish to share. Secondly, I had come to recognise, admire and respect Gabby's inner strength and resilience and I was confident that she would know, not if but when the time was right to speak. And sure enough, after a break of a few months, she arrived at a consultation ready and able to talk about some of the many disturbing experiences she had endured during childhood.

An emotional injury occurs in situations where the biologically adaptive response of primary emotion is inhibited or restricted [or denied altogether]; and, when this happens, the fulfillment of basic human needs to be loved, validated and safe, are prevented or violated. An injury of this kind has an enduring quality, experienced as *emotional pain* that burdens a person long after the event, as though a wound has not healed. ... The emotional pain can be experienced as a physical pain as well as psychological. (Harte, 2019)

Gabby's mother was an alcoholic who left Gabby's father when Gabby was 5 years old. In the first 10 years of her life, she moved house often with her mother and a growing number of siblings, usually to get away from her mother's abusive alcoholic partners. Gabby had a younger sister from her mother's first partner, another three siblings from the next partner, and a sixth child with another partner.

Gabby would often disappear from home: 'I would just go walking. I still love going for long walks to this day! I would find somewhere safe to go in the neighbourhood to get away from the arguments and violence at home.' Occasionally, the police would be called to locate her and bring her back. Gabby also found hiding places within the houses they lived in, and sought refuge there from frequent, chaotic times when things 'heated up.' She recalled how in one of the places they lived she would take refuge in the backyard toilet. Ironically, this served two purposes, one as an escape from the violence in the house but also it gave her the extra time she needed in the toilet because she suffered from chronic constipation. But alas, even there she was often disturbed by her mother banging on the door and yelling at her to get out! When I asked Gabby about the violence she had experienced, she said, 'Oh yes, my mother would often get physically violent with me. I did learn to read her and the room though, which meant I usually knew when to disappear or fade into the background. I was good at that, and still am. But after I had grown a bit, around the age of 9 or 10, I sometimes had to stand between her and the younger ones to protect them.'

Flower essence for confident social interaction: Wallflower (FES group)

I had already prescribed Wallflower essence for Gabby on a couple of occasions before the session in which she spoke about her childhood. Wallflowers often stand alone on mountainsides, with their showy bright yellow glow appearing as little splashes scattered about. Wallflower essence encourages involvement in self-assured social exchange, rather than retreat from social situations through shyness. Ironically, Gabby's acute sense of when to fade into the background had worked very much in her favour as a child! Wallflower helps us to 'stand up and stand out' while strengthening our dynamic boundaries so that we keep our core composure, without absorbing harmful energies even in volatile social situations (Wells, *Essential Flower Essence Book* p. 353).

Police removed Gabby from her home when she was 10. She ended up having to appear in court, in the presence of her mother, to say that she did not feel safe at home and did not want to go back there. Having to declare this in the intimidating surroundings of a courtroom, in the presence of her mother, who was quite a formidable figure according to Gabby, displayed real inner strength. Fortunately, court proceedings are conducted with a bit more awareness these days! Gabby was declared a ward of the state and spent the next two years in an overcrowded home with other minors. She recalled, 'I slept in the hallway for a little while before a bed of my own became available. But funnily enough, I really liked it there because I felt *safe* for the first time!' Another thing she liked about the new home was that there was a strict routine and she always knew what was going to happen next in her day; there were never any nasty surprises of the kind she had constantly endured all her life till then. However, she still had to deal with the fact that she regularly wet the bed from the age of 10 till she was 14.

At the end of two years, at around 12, she moved to another home and remained there as a ward of the state until she was 15. After that, the people in authority found her a new home with a good and caring family and she stayed with them until she was 18, when she moved into her own flat, close to where she already had a steady job in retail. As Gabby said with a smile, 'That was easy because I was very independent, having learnt the hard way to look after myself!' She met her future husband when she was 24 and they later had a son.

After Gabby's detailed and courageous revelations, we once again discussed the most appropriate flower essences for her, this time using the Flower Affinity Test—a helpful selection tool described in depth in my *Essential Flower Essence Book* (2023). The flower essences prescribed were Star of Bethlehem, Golden Ear Drops and Baby Blue Eyes. I will describe how each one related to what Gabby was going through.

Flower essence for effects of shock: Star of Bethlehem (Bach group)

Star of Bethlehem had previously been selected for Gabby on a number of occasions, serving two important purposes. Firstly, it helped her resolve her deep shock relating to the trauma she had experienced throughout her childhood, so that she didn't have to continue reliving it when triggered by events in everyday life. Star of Bethlehem is the number one, go-to flower essence for shock of all kinds. Star of Bethlehem also helped Gabby to soften psychologically so that she didn't have to use so much energy tensing in anticipation of possible triggers, or dissociating when emotional scars were activated. Because these effects of past trauma were addressed by Star of Bethlehem flower essence, the intensity of Gabby's emotional pain slowly and incrementally lessened over time. This in turn prepared her mentally and psychologically to face the vulnerability of sharing the details of her experiences. This softening was not weakness but in fact indicated that she was stronger now and more personally empowered than ever to face her demons! When we are thrown into disarray by shock—bad news, an accident, a general anaesthetic (when etheric and physical bodies become temporarily dislocated), physical or emotional violence, childbirth or other prolonged stress, even where these occurred many years ago, Star of Bethlehem flower essence helps to restore inner calm.

Negative state
Disturbed/shaken at a physical and subtle body level
Ill-effects of present and past shock and trauma

Positive state
Subtle anatomy dimensions re-aligned for healing
Release of shock and trauma
(Wells, *Essential Flower Essence Book* pp. 323–24)

Meditation for healing emotional trauma
Regular practice of meditation can work in a similar way to Star of Bethlehem, slowly helping us become more comfortable in the moment no matter what it brings up from our past. The intensity of trauma-related pain incrementally subsides, because meditation brings a state of *calm, natural ease and stillness.* I believe meditation makes us more malleable in an empowering way! The quality of pure consciousness in moments of meditation, uncontaminated by past trauma, continually shapes a better future that doesn't repeat the past. In a similar way, in emotion-focused therapy, the process of healing is therapeutically enhanced and fast-forwarded by meditation and mindfulness, enabling people to self-regulate and be more present in the moment, counteracting 'the habit of disassociation' (Harte, 2019 p. 87). This habit of dissociation had begun early in Gabby's life as a way of surviving her traumatic childhood. I believe Star of Bethlehem flower essence prepared the way for the other two remedies which Gabby was using for the first time—Baby Blue Eyes and Golden Ear Drops. Both of these are specific for the childhood issues that were now in the forefront of her mind.

Flower essence for painful memories: Golden Ear Drops (FES group)
The shape of the Golden Ear Drops flower can be likened to a teardrop, suspended in time. Painful feelings from old hurts, especially the negative emotional charge associated with childhood experiences, can become entrenched (suspended in time). Golden Ear Drops flower essence can help us gain a wiser and more comfortable perspective on

painful memories, allowing us to find resolution. Flower essences reveal only what we are ready to accept—our free will always stays intact.

Negative state
Repressed painful memories from (early) childhood
The past undermines current experiences

Positive state
'Releasing painful memories from the past' (FES)
Empowered by one's childhood experience
(Wells, *Essential Flower Essence Book* pp. 191–92)

After four weeks of taking Golden Ear Drops flower essence (along with Baby Blue Eyes and Star of Bethlehem), Gabby told me how, for the first time, without discussing it beforehand with me or anyone, she had driven by the original establishments she was placed in after the court's decision to remove her from her mother's care. She even parked outside one of them and sat there for a while, recalling how her time there had felt. She said to me, 'I felt OK about it. In fact, it was interesting to recall things about that time that I had forgotten.' In the past Gabby had always avoided the roads these places were on, barely giving them a thought when she was anywhere in the vicinity. Now, she was more comfortable with and accepting of those earlier times, and the memories were no longer so overwhelming and painful. Golden Ear Drops flower essence had enabled her to release her painful memories.

Flower essence for recovery of trust: Baby Blue Eyes (FES group)
Baby Blue Eyes helps those who have not received adequate emotional support and protection through early childhood (FES).

Negative state
Premature loss of innocence
'It's a jungle out there—you can't trust anyone.'

Positive state
'No-one's fool' but open-minded
Safe and trusting in the goodness of others
(Wells, *Essential Flower Essence Book* pp. 97–98)

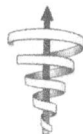

According to psychologist Lawrence Greenberg (qtd. in Lane et al., 2015), memories are malleable and constantly undergo revision. The reactivation and recalling of long-term memories during therapy—in Gabby's case while supported by me as her therapist, and by FET—renders those memories more malleable. In emotion-focused therapy (EFT), this 'initiates a re-stabilisation process termed "reconsolidation" which allows for updating of the memory' (Harte, 2019, p. 58). Golden Ear Drops and Baby Blue Eyes flower essences, used alongside elements of EFT, helped to empower Gabby throughout this process. She benefitted from the *broadening effect* of experiencing more and more positive (adaptive) and empowering emotions, and 'thus this *reprocessing* of the traumatic event [became] more than desensitising of that traumatic experience' (Harte, 2019, p. 58).

Despite Gabby's traumatic early life, she was able to identify some situations in which the *broadening effect* of positive emotions made things more bearable so that the past was no longer able to undermine the present and future in the same way. While we can categorically state that Gabby was left feeling unsafe, unworthy and unloved when the police removed her from her home at 10 years of age, the fact that she finally felt 'safe' in the 'home' where she was placed had enough of a positive (*broadening*) effect to help her adapt well to her new surroundings. Over time, after being 'treated well and fairly by the staff' and other carers, she also began to feel more valued as a person, and again this helped her to cope and adapt better to life in an institution. And much later, when she started building a family, she 'felt loved' and was able to do a great job raising her boy, giving him what she never received herself as a child. Baby Blue Eyes flower essence enabled her to find support and protection within herself and so become open to receiving from others whom she was able to discern as trustworthy.

Now, as a successful survivor, having made use of some emotion-focused therapies, Gabby's new-found freedom from the emotional pain of her past opened her mind to all sorts of possibilities. As a result, she was finally able to seek what her heart truly desired, which had become much clearer to her. This required openness and a heartfelt expression of her needs without shame or fear of emotional hostility from those close to her. The flower essence she chose and aligned with most in this process was Pink Monkeyflower, which she had never related to directly or been prescribed in previous consultations.

Flower essence for emotional courage: Pink Monkeyflower (FES group)

Pink Monkeyflower allows a person to display 'emotional transparency [and the] courage to take emotional risks with others' (FES). Fears a person may have about their true, heartfelt feelings being exposed often stem from previous emotional abuse and humiliation as children and/or teenagers, when feelings were dismissed when at their most vulnerable. With the help of Pink Monkeyflower to gently open one's heart, an individual becomes more able to comfortably express what their heart truly feels and desires in their relationships and life in general. 'They begin to experience the love and the contact [and validation] which they so desperately need and want' (FES).

Around this time, another supportive flower essence that we agreed upon was St John's Wort. It can help people when their life is expanding on an emotional, social, creative and spiritual level, and there are natural fears (many of them unconscious) about being 'out there,' taking a stand and generally experiencing life more fully. Gabby's expansive plans going forward would inevitably take her into the unknown and out of her comfort zone, partly because they would impact significantly on those close to her. But she believed wholeheartedly, 'It's my time now!' No-one could possibly argue about that!

Flower essence for freedom from fear: St John's Wort (FES group)

One aspect of the doctrine of signatures of the St John's Wort plant relates to the way a vulnerability in humans (in this case being too open and exposed) corresponds to a particular strength in a plant—in this case, St John's Wort's unique receptivity to the sun's healing rays. St John's Wort can help us transform over-exposed openness into a dynamic capacity to soak up healing energies from our surroundings. This protective quality was recognised by the ancient Greeks, who believed that the fragrance of St John's Wort could repel evil spirits. Christian priests in the Middle Ages continued the tradition, performing exorcisms using the plant, which they associated with St John the Baptist. St John's Wort should be considered when we feel exposed on a subtle level. It is extremely useful for those experiencing a feeling of vulnerability or 'thin skin' for no apparent reason. Also, St John's Wort may help us feel more secure during psychoanalysis or regression therapies, when deeply entrenched fears may surface.

Negative state
Feeling vulnerable; 'deep fears' (FES)
Disturbed sleep/dreams (FES)

Positive state
Confident and secure
Sunny disposition
(Wells, *Essential Flower Essence Book* pp. 301–02)

For Gabby this flower essence was a beautiful follow-on from Baby Blue Eyes. Her now-restored belief and trust in life became a catalyst that enabled her to venture out into the world as she never had before.

As we have described many times in this book, the *broadening effect* of positive emotion can enhance creativity, expand people's repertoire of desired actions, increase their openness to new experiences, and 'widen peoples' outlooks in ways that, little by little, beneficially reshape who they are' (Frederickson & Kurtz, 2001 p. 36). Up until now, Gabby had never looked too far ahead and always remained available to those who needed her—her son, partner, clients in her small business and others she came across in life. This is admirable but for the first time she was now looking more directly at what she really desired for herself and how she might go about manifesting this, without impacting negatively on her loved ones and those who depended on her. The life she always desired had begun.

Case study: My heart's desire ...

As mentioned earlier, when I was 8 years old, a doctor diagnosed a heart murmur and stated that at some stage later in life I would most likely need a heart valve replacement. Almost half a century later at 51 years of age, while playing tennis I collapsed, and tests at the hospital emergency department confirmed the earlier prediction. My aortic valve was 85% obstructed—such a severe a diagnosis it prompted the doctor to say, 'Wrap yourself up in cotton wool until you see the cardiac specialist on Monday.' It was late Friday afternoon so I spent the weekend feeling nervous but philosophical while pondering all the possibilities.

On a few occasions in the past, when feeling extremely challenged, or in a life-threatening situation as was the case this time, I had taken the Australian Bush Flower essence Waratah, which helped me to face my issues and remain proactive in working through them. In these situations I often use the expression, 'Feel the fear in one hand, and take action with the other.' The doctor had rightly sounded the alarm, recognising that open heart surgery would almost certainly be necessary asap to replace my damaged heart valve. I started taking Waratah as soon as I got home from the hospital. Fortunately, my teenage son and daughter were otherwise occupied that weekend, so I was able to meditate without interruption. Meditation has always helped me to ground myself and remain mindful of my needs, values and life purpose, while helping me to accept and deal with anxiety. At that moment, issues of life and death and my mortality were definitely in the forefront of my mind.

Flower essence for responding to crisis: Waratah (Aus Bush group)

Waratah flower essence is used to help *stir our survival instincts* when we are facing a life crisis. The Waratah flower is very important in Aboriginal culture, folklore and legends which tell the stories of individuals who survive crises, *ordeals and life challenges*, becoming stronger through the development of *courage, faith and endurance.*

Negative state
Hopelessness and utter despair (Ian White)
In crisis and unable to respond

Positive state
'Enhancement of survival skills' (Ian White)
Active and composed in a crisis
(Wells, *Essential Flower Essence Book* pp. 356–57)

The regular experience of *calm, natural ease and stillness* during meditation flows into the rest of your day, making it especially helpful when experiencing difficulty. It helps reduce anxiety and fear during stressful times, so that you can stay grounded and focused on the job at hand (something I desperately needed when faced with the prospect of heart surgery!) Over that weekend, I was able to clarify in my mind what I desired in terms of my wellbeing and more specifically, the areas where I would not compromise. One thing I was very clear about was that I did not want to be dependent on medication. For example, I did not want to take blood thinning medication for the rest of my life, which would be necessary if I were given an artificial replacement valve. I intend no disrespect to those who have *correctly*, for many important reasons, chosen to use such medication. It is just that, when it comes to *my* health, I do it my way, using the best information I can obtain as it applies to *my* situation, and so far that has worked for me! So, an artificial valve was not an option, but beyond this I couldn't make many decisions until I had spoken with the cardiac specialist. So I remained clear and focused on my vision of the life I desired after surgery.

Monday's appointment with the specialist came around and he confirmed that I would need a valve replacement. I told him I would prefer not to have an artificial valve and asked about the possibility of using biological tissue from pig or cow. His response was, 'Let's see how the angiogram goes—you're booked for two days from now.' I went away determined to learn more! I knew that a biological tissue valve typically lasts around 12–15 years before a replacement is required, and asked myself, 'Do I really want to go through open-heart surgery again when I am older if I can in any way avoid it?' Also, I knew that blood-thinning medication is often required for a period after this surgery. Despite my many questions and niggling fears, I had already started to feel more positive and motivated about my predicament. I also felt somewhat comforted knowing I had more options than I first thought, and that my specialist was open to discussing them.

Buoyed by this positivity, I spent until the early hours of the morning online, researching and obtaining as much information as possible about my best options. I managed to remain *positive* and persevered despite having moments of feeling terrified about the impending surgery. I was able to take my own advice—I felt the fear in one hand and took action with the other. My determination came from being clear about my *personal values* regarding finding alternatives to being dependent on medication, and keeping the focus primarily on my quality of life going forward. I was able to keep my *mind open* to all possibilities. This was another example of the *broadening effect* of positive emotions, which facilitates creative responses (Ziv, 1976) and problem solving (Isen et al., 1987). I was able to dive in, despite my fears, and use lateral (creative) thinking and research to pursue my goal of the best possible outcome. At about 3.00 am, I came across an article about Arnold Schwarzenegger (thanks Arnie!), which described how he had undergone a form of heart valve replacement surgery known as the Ross Procedure, which uses human tissue, does not require ongoing blood-thinning medication, and for most patients needs no re-intervention for over 20 years. The next morning I rang my cardiac specialist and said, 'Have you heard of the Ross Procedure?' There was a pause and he replied, 'Ah, well, I have heard about it … but let's wait for the test results.' Next morning after the angiogram, as I drowsily surfaced from the anaesthetic, the specialist leaned over me and said enthusiastically, 'The rest of your heart and blood vessels are in good condition, so you are a prime candidate for the Ross Procedure, and guess what? The only surgeon in Australia who does the operation practises right here in Melbourne!'

I could hear that he was happy for me, and I also appreciated that he had obviously done a fair bit of homework in the last 24 hours! The surgeon's location may have been fortuitous, but I have no doubt that the fact that I came across the Ross Procedure, which aligned with my goals and my personal values was not just luck! My discovery of the procedure was made possible because I remained in a positive frame of mind despite my fears, and this enabled me to do the research and be creative in my thinking. I always stayed hopeful.

The Ross Procedure takes six or seven hours, and for this reason it is usually reserved for younger people, as such a long operation involves some risk for those over 50, especially if they have other health issues. Being 51 at the time, I had to convince the appropriately cautious surgeon of my good health. 'I don't smoke, I drink alcohol once a year on Christmas day, my diet and lifestyle are very healthy, I keep fit, and I'm a naturopath who practises what he preaches. I will be your star patient!' Finally, after he had physically examined me, he agreed to perform the operation. However, my excitement subsided when he told me he was going away for a four week holiday and would operate after he got back. I didn't have enough cotton wool to keep myself wrapped up for that long! I pleaded with him (it was worth a try!): 'Is there any chance you could do it before you go away?' This was on Monday morning. He replied, 'I leave on Friday. I could possibly do it this Wednesday if I can get hold of a pulmonary valve from a deceased donor by then—but that's not likely to happen.' However, to his surprise, he was able to obtain a valve. I was operated on, successfully, on Wednesday morning.

I was able to remain positive, focused and calm throughout my dealings with the specialist and the surgeon with the help of FET and meditation. Sure, there was some anxiety, but I was able to manage it and give myself the best chance of getting what I desired. And 17 years on, according to the surgeon my heart and the replacement valve are in great condition and have not deteriorated since the operation— something he has not witnessed before and always seems surprised about when he studies my echocardiogram. At some point during each annual appointment he says, 'What do you do again Mark?' I answer, 'I work as a naturopath and counsellor,' and he usually replies, 'Whatever you're doing, keep doing it!'

IMPEDIMENTS TO EMOTIONAL EXPRESSION

Returning to the sailboat image we used earlier, you could say that people think about their emotions the way a captain thinks about the ship's compass. What does the captain think when the compass indicates that the boat is heading in an undesired direction? Do they believe that changing the boat's course will change the feedback from the compass? Or do they think their actions will make no difference? Can I change my feelings or am I at their mercy? Does the captain believe that feedback showing the boat is going the wrong way proves that they are not worthy to be a sailor? Does the captain think that this type of feedback should be avoided? A captain who believes that unfavourable feedback from the compass is unacceptable may deliberately ignore it and live in denial. If the captain believes they can't change the compass feedback or their emotions OR ignores them, they miss out on the opportunity to turn the boat in the desired direction when it has been diverted (Gandhiplein 16).

BELIEFS ABOUT THE ACCEPTABILITY OF EMOTIONS

Many people have beliefs about emotions that operate outside conscious awareness and relate to what kinds of emotional expression are deemed appropriate and acceptable by family, religious authorities or society in general. Beliefs about the unacceptability of experiencing or expressing 'negative' thoughts and emotions may play a key role in the development and maintenance of clinical problems (Surawy et al., 1995) and can be associated with worse prognoses and treatment outcomes (Corstorphine, 2006). Beliefs about the unacceptability of emotions can be perceived as dysfunctional assumptions associated with a range of different problems such as depression (Cramer et al., 2005), eating disorders (Corstorphine, 2006), post-traumatic stress disorder (Ehlers & Clark, 2000), and borderline personality disorder (Linehan, 1993). Throughout this book I have described the negative consequences for mental and physical health of beliefs that lead to the avoidance of emotions. Growing up in an environment where the expression of difficult or negative feelings is avoided, discouraged, 'medicated' or seen as inappropriate according to gender, can have lasting consequences.

Case study: Emotions and gender

In my book, *Embracing the Gift of High Sensitivity* (2021), I describe how 'Sylvia,' a highly sensitive client, reflects on the impact of her upbringing and how, in her family, certain emotions and behaviours were discouraged and others encouraged according to gender. 'As a girl growing up in a large family it was fine for me to become teary or over-excited and/or emotional about things … but if I displayed anger or aggro, I was quickly put in my place for not behaving like a proper little lady, or worse, I'd get the anger thrown back at me in spades! … My brothers, however, would often hurl abuse, sometimes even break things in a rage … and that was just seen as boys being boys! Later in life, especially when I had young children, I found it extremely difficult to deal with my intense emotional reactions. My anxiety levels became unbearable. I was totally overwhelmed for a time there and was not coping until I decided to seek help. I held on to anger, too … I just didn't know how to deal with it' (p. 110).

During Sylvia's upbringing, much of her anger became repressed. I have described previously how anger, like all emotion, can be incredibly useful and informative. Dr Elaine Aron (1997) tells us that feelings of anger are a signal that you need to 'stand up for yourself or leave.' It can be an emotion we fear because by expressing anger we often get anger back—as Sylvia did, 'in spades'!

Other problems can also arise when expression of certain emotions is expected as part of acceptable 'womanly' or 'manly' behaviour. In

Sylvia's family her hyper-excited, or teary, sad emotions were condoned, and so were her brothers' aggressive or angry behaviours. Aron (2001 p. 82) tells us that 'unlike the boys, if [girls] display some overarousal or emotion, they are doing what is [stereotypically] expected of them.'

Beliefs about the malleability of emotions

Throughout this book we have described the *broadening effect* of positive emotion, enabled by FET, meditation and emotion-focused therapies. However, many people strongly believe that they cannot change their emotions, no matter how hard they try, and are thus not motivated to attempt emotional self-regulation. I am reminded of a news story about a prison officer who took part in an elaborate conspiracy with criminals outside the prison system to enable a prisoner to escape from jail. The escapee was eventually caught, and the prison officer's involvement was revealed. At the trial, she was asked why she aided the prisoner in such a crime. She replied, 'Because I had fallen in love with him,' with the implication that her actions were therefore outside of her control, and she had no choice! (Not surprisingly, that defence didn't stand up too well in court.) By contrast, if people believe that emotions can be changed, they will actively attempt to emotionally self-regulate.

As we have seen, the *broadening effect* experienced after taking flower essences or through practising meditation motivates people so that the next time they experience negative emotions they are more self-assured, more proactive and more likely to display resilience. My experience with Willow flower essence described earlier is a good example.

The sailboat: Returning to the sailboat image, a person who believes that there is nothing they can do to change emotions is like a captain who believes they can have no influence over the feedback from the compass and perceive themselves as powerless. Obviously, when the boat is steered in a different direction, the feedback from the compass will automatically change, and in the same way, emotions can be changed by acknowledging them and taking action. The captain has power to change the feedback from the compass by turning the wheel of the boat. A captain who believes that their actions can change the feedback from the compass uses the compass as it is intended: as a navigational aid designed to help them adjust the course of the journey when needed. (Gandhiplein 16)

Addressing unhelpful beliefs about emotions is a fundamental component of many therapies, most of which use psychoeducation and teach clients to question their existing judgments and beliefs. The idea is that by critically examining emotional beliefs, their impact can be reduced. Practitioners help clients to examine the long-term consequences of their assumptions, consider how assumptions can become self-fulfilling, and identify the advantages and disadvantages of holding onto these assumptions.

I spoke previously of a client and his relationship with anger. He described to me how his wife would often 'get angry and show no control of herself.' At these times he would clam up (later admitting to himself that this was a form of passive aggression) and say to his wife, 'Please control yourself, otherwise I am not going to discuss this with you.' You can imagine how this inflamed the situation and how she felt. My client eventually recognised the part he was playing in the dynamic with his wife. She was expressing anger and frustration for two people because he was unable to recognise, acknowledge and express it for himself. He had the belief (reinforced by his upbringing) that anger shouldn't be overtly expressed. Through psychoeducation, he came to the realisation that this belief also protected him from acknowledging and expressing anger, about which he felt very fearful.

Taking Scarlet Monkeyflower flower essence helped him to become more comfortable with his anger, and more able to stay with it as it began to lose its negative impact on him. He then began to feel less threatened when his wife expressed anger, and eventually was able to feel and express some appropriate amount of his own anger and frustration, and still remain adequately self-regulated. He told me, 'We are now able to have good discussions, sometimes a little heated but they don't get out of hand anymore.' He no longer identified with or was subordinate to his family's belief that any overt expression of anger was inappropriate, would inevitably escalate out of control, and served no purpose.

Meditation-based therapies reduce the impact of dysfunctional beliefs by enabling people to observe them rather than accept them as truth—in the same way they observe their emotions as just part of their whole Self. Rather than challenging irrational beliefs about emotions, meditation practice involves reducing over-identification with these beliefs. Then we learn to see the difference between beliefs and reality.

UNCONSCIOUS AVOIDANCE OF DEEP EMOTION

> The first layer we encounter in the unconscious is what Jung called the shadow, usually those parts of ourselves we don't like, don't know, or don't want to know. The shadow can be repressed in us like a cancer or projected outward onto others as qualities we dislike most in a person or group. The negative shadow can present us with a shortcoming to be overcome. The positive can show us a meaningful part of ourselves we should recognise and live out. Either way it's a tricky element to deal with as Jung himself knew. (Dunne, 2015, p. 106)

'*The shadow can be repressed in us like a cancer or projected outward onto others as qualities we dislike most in a person or group.*' Carl Jung saw our shadow side as being made up of repressed (unconscious) qualities we don't like about ourselves, which we often project outward onto others. Studying one's shadow side can be life-changing for someone who is dedicated to personal growth. The study of the shadow is as personally confronting as it gets—just as confronting as looking at our own illness to inform us about what we might be projecting onto our bodies and other external factors such as pathogens, as causes of our illness.

Flower essence for Self-awareness: Black Eyed Susan (FES group)

Black Eyed Susan's flower confronts with its black central zone projecting outward at you from the striking contrast of its yellow surrounds. You can try but you can't avoid it! Black Eyed Susan flower essence is a powerful catalyst to help us confront certain aspects of our personality which may have been too uncomfortable to face until now. In colour therapy, yellow is associated with the intellect, and in those who can benefit from Black Eyed Susan essence, it is the intellect that edits and represses what a person has adjudged to be his/her 'darker' emotions— the *shadow side* signified by the flower's black centre.

Negative state
Repressed and mentally 'edited' feelings
'Festering' emotion—'emotional boils'

Positive state
Self-awareness through 'penetrating insight' (FES)
Opening the doors to our full potential
(Wells, *Essential Flower Essence Book* p. 108)

When we perceive emotion as something negative that must be hidden, this belief can unconsciously, and often malignantly, influence our perception of the world and others. Anger, selfishness, desire, greed, cowardice—all of these and more make up the shadow self. The history of human beings is riddled with atrocities and hateful acts that have occurred because of people's unconscious projections of their shadow aspects onto others. Hate crimes are an example of this.

Jung was deeply interested in the nature and content of the shadow and in the importance of integrating those things we don't want and don't like about ourselves. He saw that the inability to examine our shadow components prevents us from perceiving our own deep emotions and primal instincts, and so prevents us from fully understanding our own motivations and behaviours.

'The knowledge of the heart is in no book and is not
to be found in the mouth of any teacher, but grows out of you
like the green seed from the dark earth.'

(Jung, *The Red Book*)

In summary, the benefits of working with your shadow side are:

- *Self-awareness*: Recognising hidden aspects of yourself.
- *Emotional resilience*: Managing and understanding emotions.
- *Personal growth*: Embracing all parts of yourself to live more authentically.
- *Improved relationships*: Understanding your shadow can enhance empathy and connection with others. (centreofexcellence.com)

Fear of the intensity of emotions

Many people have a fear of how intense their emotional reactions to life circumstances could become. A common fear is that we won't be able to control emotions once we allow them to be present, and that we could be overwhelmed by them and do something we regret. We may have grown up in a household in which this overwhelm is precisely what happened on a regular basis, or we ourselves might have lost the plot at times of intense emotion. This fear creates more stress, and at the same time, intense emotions continually bottled up become even more extreme. As we described earlier, internalisation of strong emotion through suppression requires enormous conscious and unconscious self-regulatory resources that ultimately become exhausted. When this point is reached, many people become completely overwhelmed and collapse, or worse, erupt violently, which confirms their fear of emotion, and so a vicious cycle is established or reinforced. This was the case for the man I described earlier for whom I prescribed Scarlet Monkeyflower flower essence, who had previously been unable to connect with and recognise his own anger, which was manifesting as passive aggression in his relationship with his wife. A fear of intense feelings can cause people to actively suppress or avoid emotions. All the Monkeyflower flower essences help us to address our fear of fully experiencing and expressing different kinds of intense emotion:

- **Scarlet Monkeyflower:** Awareness and fear of anger and 'heated' emotion in oneself and others.
- **Sticky Monkeyflower:** Fear of intense feelings associated with intimacy and sensuality.
- **Mimulus (common yellow monkeyflower):** Fear/anticipatory anxiety around speaking and standing up for oneself in everyday life.
- **Pink Monkeyflower:** Fear of engaging with and exposing one's true and heartfelt feelings.
- **Purple Monkeyflower:** Fear of intense spiritual experience, and inabilitiy to trust in one's higher Self.

The regular practice of meditation enables us to stay present to our emotions, even intense ones, long enough to establish a different relationship with them. We get better at accepting them and observing them as just a part of who we are. Being less attached to them, they are therefore 'disarmed' and no longer overwhelm or take us over. They can then inform and provide us with important insights into what is happening in our lives and around us.

In summary, although avoidance of intense feelings may result in short-term relief, it will not help in the long run and creates further problems. A constant and uneasy fear remains, that emotions will eventually take over in some dramatic way—and in fact, by the time these pent-up feelings are finally released it can seem as if the metaphorical floodgates have opened! Then your self-fulfilling prophecy—'I was right, look what happens when I let go!'—comes to fruition.

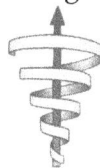

'Stuck' in surface emotion

Rather than avoiding deeper emotions, experiencing them fully and expressing them teaches us that although they can be painful, with time and practice they also become more bearable and easier to regulate. Meditation, FET and EFT can fast-forward this process. For example, when people who find it very uncomfortable and difficult to cry (and try to keep a stiff upper lip or laugh it off) finally weep, they *don't* remain in a sobbing heap forever, as they had previously expected. In fact, they usually feel relief and become more secure in themselves, coming to the realisation that their fears were not justified. However, as we have seen throughout this book, this process can be complicated, so guidance is required. People are often not aware of their primary underlying feelings, as described in the section on adaptive and maladaptive emotions, and can remain stuck in experiencing superficial (secondary) emotions. Here is a story told to me by a Traditional Chinese Medicine practitioner, which describes this situation:

> *In ancient China, there was once an emperor who ruled during a peaceful time, when his people were settled and content. And yet, the emperor was an intense worrier. Though he had no conflicts to deal with, he ruminated over petty things, making mountains out of molehills, and his life was miserable. His mental and physical health was suffering as a consequence, so his advisors summoned the most renowned physician in China to attend him. At his first session, it wasn't long before the emperor stormed out, telling his advisors, 'All he did was tease and provoke me—he didn't even prescribe any medicine!' After a few days, the emperor's advisors managed to get him to consult the physician again, but again, the emperor stormed out halfway through the meeting, even more outraged, saying, 'He takes pleasure in annoying and infuriating me!' At this point, the emperor's health did not seem to be improving, and he was even more irritable than usual, while still being tormented by worry. His advisors had their work cut out to convince him to consult the physician again, but after promising that if he would give it one more try, they would not trouble him further, he reluctantly agreed. This time, the physician succeeded in sending the emperor into a monumental rage— he smashed furniture and threw it out the windows; he hurled unsecured objects around the palace, narrowly missing his advisors who were collectively running for cover! But when he finally settled down, he had to admit that he hadn't felt this good in years.*

As my TCM practitioner friend informed me, it is situations such as this that gave rise to the expression, 'You need to vent your spleen!' In TCM, overthinking/rumination causing worry can be the negative effect of an imbalance in the stomach/spleen meridian. The positive effect of a balanced stomach/spleen meridian is *healthy reflection, insight* and *clear thinking*. I have described in the previous section on repressed emotion in physical illness how TCM regards all emotions as equally important; an unhealthy state arises when the flow of differing emotions stops or is bypassed, and we get stuck in experiencing one emotion. In this case, the emperor was stuck in worry and rumination and was unable to allow the flow to move on into other feelings. TCM recommends that when we get stuck in a feeling, it can help to go *backwards* through the cycle of emotions (Fig. 10) to get feelings flowing *forwards* again. In the case of the emperor's worry, the imperial physician worked on stirring up—going *backwards* and engaging with—the emperor's underlying and unexpressed anger/frustration. By engaging with and venting frustration, which is two steps *backwards* in the TCM emotions cycle and is associated with the liver/gall/bladder meridian, the cycle was able to start flowing *forwards* again, without getting stuck in excessive worry and rumination. It's like the situation where we dig a hole for ourselves by spinning the wheels of a vehicle and get bogged in mud or sand. If we don't have anyone to tow us out, we can reverse slightly back up the side of the hole and take a speedy run out of the stuck place, so that *forward momentum* frees us.

Figure 10: How emotions and organs are connected in TCM

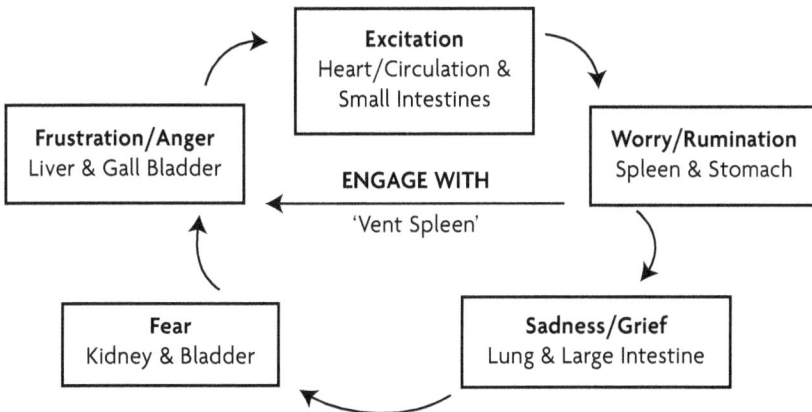

Disclosing and sharing painful emotions in a safe environment can create a sense of trust in a relationship. Expressing emotions that may have been hidden can show that one feels safe enough to disclose deeply personal information. During my single parenting time, I recall how my two teenagers would come home after a tough day at school, or after a game of basketball in which they felt they played badly, or when they were just in a passing bad mood about life in general. At those times, all the unexpressed feelings they'd held in while with their peers and out in public would finally surface once they got home—often to be dumped on me! Anything I said would be met with ire, and they would tell me what a stupid ****** I was. I learnt to do my best to just engage with them through active listening and let their high emotional state run its course—easier said than done! A good friend often commented at the time, 'Isn't that great! They obviously feel really safe with you'—just as the emperor in the story finally felt safe with his physician! I responded by telling her that in the middle of being used as a verbal and emotional punching bag it's hard to step back and say to yourself, 'Isn't this lovely that my kids feel safe enough to call me a stupid ******!!' Ultimately, it is therapeutic for them to have someone that they can share their most painful (usually hidden) emotions with, while you do your best to help them learn to better self-regulate and grow. If you can lead by example and learn to better regulate yourself during these intense emotional exchanges, it can all pay off in the end; you develop great trust in each other as years go by. My kids are much nicer to me now!

Expressing superficial emotion to avoid deeper emotion

On the surface, one may think that it is always good to talk about your feelings/emotions. In principle that's a good philosophy and certainly way better than always keeping a stiff upper lip! However, there are questions it's wise to ask yourself: What exactly are the emotions I am expressing? Are they emotions that are only *on the surface*, or that I think others can tolerate? Am I expressing only those emotions that are socially acceptable according to my belief system? If this is the case, ask yourself: Do I engage in superficial emotionality to avoid expressing deeper and more uncomfortable emotions? A simple example may be a client who comes to you who has had to drive through peak hour traffic and is running late. They enter the consultation room irritated, frustrated and angry, and because they strongly believe that talking about an emotion will reduce its intensity they verbally express their anger and frustration as a way to get rid of these feelings. But we know these very recent feelings are superficial and the client, with guidance, will settle down in a few minutes and commence talking about deeper, more significant, emotions they are experiencing.

Just because someone is *talking* about emotions doesn't necessarily mean they are *feeling* that deeper layer that belongs to their primary emotional response to what is happening! Often, a person avoids experiencing difficult emotions and tries to reduce them by compulsively talking about other feelings. For instance, after experiencing a negative emotional event, a person, now in a hyper-emotional state, immediately calls a friend to 'offload' and share their experience in the hope that this will make the negative feeling go away. Instead of taking some time to genuinely connect to the experience and be more aware of the deep emotion it has triggered, the person immediately jumps into problem-solving with the help of their compliant friend, getting rid of negative feeling as quickly as possible. The friend who is listening to the story says the right things to reduce negative feelings but this will only help in the short term.

Flower essence for genuine emotional expression: Fuchsia (FES group)

As described earlier, Fuchsia flower essence has been very helpful to clients who are in an alternating cycle of being hyper-emotional, then hypo-emotional, avoiding fully experiencing deeper emotions. This flower essence has the ability to ground people and allow them to embrace their true feelings (Wells, *Essential Flower Essence Book* p.185).

Negative state
Psychosomatic symptoms resulting from emotional repression (FES)
'False states of emotionality' (FES); 'over the top' reactions

Positive state
Deep awareness / Self-understanding
Genuine (primary) emotional expression; grounded

EMOTIONAL VOCABULARY

If people have difficulty identifying and labelling their emotions (Vine & Aldao, 2014), it affects their ability to relate directly with them and so lessens their awareness and ability to understand which emotions need to be regulated. Even if you have some sense of your feelings, if you don't have the words to articulate or 'flesh them out,' those feelings can easily remain hidden. And further, the frustration felt at not being able to find the right words creates another impediment to recognising deeper, primary emotions and/or increases the level and intensity of emotion needing to be regulated. Helping clients expand their emotional vocabulary can be an important step in increasing their emotional regulation skills and ability to express emotion.

Flower essence for finding your voice: Cosmos (FES group)

Cosmos helps people who are finding it hard to express their thoughts and feelings, or who verbalise in a disordered or confused way. They may feel frustrated in their ability to clearly articulate opinions on certain issues that are important to them. Cosmos flower essence has helped many of my clients to 'find their voice.' Cosmos's deep red-purple flower immediately commands attention; you cannot help but notice it. It 'speaks' to you with clarity and colour and these extrovert qualities can help you unravel and externalise what you really *feel* inside. Some people even find the flower's colour a 'bit rich' when confronted by its clear and uncompromising, honest expression.

Negative state
'Overwhelmed by too many ideas' (FES)
Emotionally inarticulate—overexcited or erratic speech

Positive state
Speaking and living your heartfelt truth
Emotionally articulate (FES)—coherent speech
(Wells, *Essential Flower Essence Book* p. 155)

Writing to express feelings

Writer and psychotherapist Dennis Palumbo says: 'Initially, when you start writing, or at least when I started writing, you think the reward is, wow! It'll be so great to see my words on screen, to see my name on screen. ... [But over time] what happens—and it's a subtle change ... is the gratification becomes personal ... the process of writing becomes its own reward ... you tell the story the way you want to tell the story' (Creative Mind).

There are great benefits to be got from written expression of one's emotions but as with all experience of deep feelings it may initially be uncomfortable. Over time, it gets easier and can form a very effective outlet, especially when other avenues are not available. Pennebaker and

Beall (1986) found that writing about feelings associated with a traumatic event brought increased arousal on the first day, but decreased arousal on three consecutive days afterwards. People should be aware that the benefits of self-expressive writing develop over time. Although some people do gain immediate benefits, written disclosure of emotions is not a 'quick fix.'

> **The sailboat:** In the sailboat metaphor, an example of written expression of emotions would be the captain using the feedback from the compass to make notes in his logbook. The captain uses his logbook to write down the most important compass observations and to respond to questions such as 'What did the feedback from the compass teach me about the current part of my journey?' 'According to the compass, is my boat sailing on track?' (Gandhiplein 16)

In my practice, I have found that occasionally when commencing taking flower essences, clients become more aware of the very emotions or attitudes they are hoping to manage, change, and/or improve. This increased awareness, accompanied by increased arousal, is also a sign that the remedy is a good match, and the person can be assured of feeling much better over the next few days. This heightened response is not essential, and usually, increased arousal *doesn't* occur—rather, there is a raised general awareness and steady improvement.

An initial, strong, felt sense of increased arousal is common and important in EFT and can also sometimes be experienced in meditation and other therapies. When very anxious people start meditating for the first time, they may initially experience a heightened awareness of their anxiety/fear. After all, better awareness and insight is the aim, and as we described above, you cannot self-regulate something you have not identified. With a little support, hyper-awareness of this kind usually subsides quickly, and meditation enables better self-regulation and acceptance of anxiety, as its intensity and negative impact subsides. In EFT one must deal with high emotional arousal levels at the beginning of therapy as part of processing past emotionally painful trauma. This process is therapeutically enhanced by meditation and mindfulness practices that help people to stay present to their emotions rather than dissociating. In natural therapy professions such as naturopathy, homeopathy, osteopathy etc. some have called this short-lived initial heightened awareness of symptoms a 'healing crisis,' and see it as a good sign. (I want to stress once again that it doesn't always occur, but is experienced by a small minority.)

In my observation of the health and healing professions overall, including in my own practice, I have found that an over-emphasis and intense focus by a client on their mental or emotional symptoms can easily create what appears to be a healing crisis but is not, and this can be further exacerbated if the therapist also misinterprets it. This self-generated focus to the point of total distraction for the client is *not* a healing crisis and more often indicates that the flower essence or therapy is not having the impact required, and that counselling is the best course of action for the time being. Once a client has a better understanding and awareness of their own process they can engage better in emotional self-regulation, and at this stage, another flower essence can be considered.

Pennebaker (1990) suggest that 'repeatedly confronting an upsetting experience allows for a less emotionally laden assessment of its meaning and impact' (p. 106). Repeated self-reflection is a way to expose oneself to an emotion and thereby reduce its negative impact incrementally, through a form of 'de-sensitising' (see Gabby's case with Star of Bethlehem). In meditation, a person learns to sit and 'be with' their anxiety until they develop a different relationship with it, and in this way it loses its negative impact on them. They reach a point where their anxiety is perceived very differently, as something separate from *Self*. Anxiety loses its hold and they get a better grip on Self!

Music to express feelings

Over the ages music has often been described as the 'language of the emotions.' Modern research also shows that listeners perceive music as being expressive of emotions (for a review, see Gabrielsson & Juslin, 2003). We have all experienced how performers of music—singers, bands and orchestras—can communicate emotions. In a meta-analysis of 41 studies, Justin and Laukka (2003) showed that professional performers are able to communicate five emotions (happiness, anger, sadness, fear, tenderness) to listeners as accurately as through facial and verbal expression. For instance, just as people who are happy tend to talk faster, happy music is characterised by a higher tempo. Likewise, just as the expression of sadness is characterised by a softer voice, sad music tends to have a lower sound level. One may express an emotion by creating music that mimics the characteristics of that emotion. For many of us who don't create music, our listening selection may match the feelings we are currently experiencing, providing an avenue of expression. I sometimes reach for ACDC's hard rock when I feel frustrated and irritated and need to vent! Or when I need to lift my spirits, I play cheerful music to express and experience more joy.

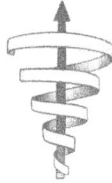

My intent for this book has been to hold up a holistic lens that brings into focus a multidimensional view of the Self in all its aspects, including our vulnerabilities and strengths and our unlimited possibilities. Using practical and natural therapies such as flower essence, meditation, and emotion-focused therapies, we can heal and harness our emotional nature to rise like a phoenix from the ashes and realise our full, innate, and unconditional potential.

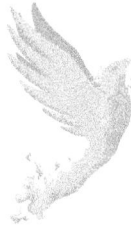

ABOUT THE AUTHOR

Mark has four decades of experience in private practice as a naturopath and counsellor in Melbourne, Australia, where prior to graduating in Naturopathy, he completed a Biological Science degree (majoring in Genetics and Zoology) at La Trobe Uni. He then worked in Special Education for five years at Kew Cottages Special School.

While maintaining a practice and caring for his two children, Mark lectured at the Southern School of Natural Therapies in Melbourne for 14 years, completed a Postgraduate Diploma in Qualitative Research and conducted formal research into Rescue Remedy™ at Victoria University. He has published six books on natural therapies, and completed his Master of Social Science (Counselling) at Swinburne University, where his placement experience was as a family counsellor and co-facilitator of mindfulness meditation groups as part of the Geelong Hospital Chronic Pain Management programme. He also completed a Stillness

Meditation Therapy teacher training course. Mark's naturopathic 'tools of trade' are drawn from multiple health modalities in which he has expertise, including homeopathy, flower essence therapy, herbal medicine, iridology, counselling, psychotherapy and emotion-focused therapy, and meditation therapy. Over the years he has treated thousands of clients with many different health issues, and with much success.

As a therapist, Mark's approach is above all else holistic, and his empathic understanding supports and comforts his clients. He identifies the root causes of their physical health issues. He then draws on his expertise and decades of experience in multiple health modalities to enable clients to attain physical and emotional health and wellbeing.

Mark has a special interest in the health of highly sensitive persons (HSPs). As an HSP himself, he gains great satisfaction from assisting other HSPs, both adults and children, to live physically and mentally healthy, contented, and productive lives that make room for their sensitivity and respect their depth of feeling and perception.

Other books by Mark Wells

The Bach Flowers Today. Melbourne: Mark Wells, 2013.

Embracing the Gift of High Sensitivity: A Guide to Living Joyfully. Melbourne: Brolga Publishing, 2021.

The Essential Flower Essence Book: Flower Essences for Living, Healing, Personal Growth and Blossoming. Melbourne: HSP Health, 2023.

Twelve Dynamic Elements of Good Health: The Tissue Salts. Melbourne: Mark Wells, 2016.

Simon, A. & Wells, M. *The Cosmos in the Cauldron: Combining the Wisdom of Astrology and the Innate Intelligence of Plants and Minerals to Heal and Grow.* Melbourne: Wells Naturopathic Centre, 2019.

RESOURCES
Flower Essence Therapy (FET):
Mark Wells BSc. ND. MSocSc.
Naturopath & Counsellor, Teacher/Lecturer and Author
PO Box 79 Kew East
VIC 3102, Australia
+ 61 409 985 970
email: wellsmark1313@gmail.com
website: hsphealth.com.au
HSP Health
439 Riversdale Road, Hawthorn East
VIC 3123, Australia

Australian Bush Flower Essences (AUS):
45 Booralie Road, Terrey Hills
NSW 2084, Australia
+61 2 9450 1388
email: info@ausflowers.com.au
website: ausflowers.com.au

Bach Flower Remedies:
Nelsons
Nelsons House, 83 Parkside, Wimbledon
London SW19 5LP
+44 (0)20 8780 4240
website: nelsons.com

Flower Essence Services (FES):
PO Box 1769 Nevada City
CA 95959
(800) 548-0075
email: mail@fesflowers.com
website: fesflowers.com
Contact for local distributor

Emotion-Focused Therapy (EFT):
Australian Institute of Emotion Focused Therapy (AIEFT)
Level 1, 16A Toorak Rd, South Yarra
VIC 3141, Australia

REFERENCES

Alberts, H., Schneider, F., & Martijn, C. (2012). Dealing efficiently with emotions: Acceptance-based coping with negative emotions requires fewer resources than suppression. *Cognition and Emotion*, *26*(5), 863–870. doi.org/10.1080/02699931.2011.625402

Allen, L. B., McHugh, R. K., & Barlow, D. H. (2008). Emotional disorders: A unified protocol. In D. H. Barlow (Ed.), *Clinical handbook of psychological disorders: A step-by-step treatment manual* (pp. 216–249). New York: Guilford Press.

Arntz, A., Lancee, J., & Morina, N. (2017). Imagery rescripting as a clinical intervention for aversive memories: A meta-analysis. *Journal of Behavior Therapy and Experimental Psychiatry*, 55, 6–15. doi:10.1016/j.jbtep.2016.11.003

Aron, E. (1997). *The highly sensitive person: How to thrive when the world overwhelms you.* Portland: Broadway Books.

Aron, E. (2001). *The highly sensitive person in love: Understanding and managing relationships when the world overwhelms you.* Harmony Books.

Aviezer, H., Trope, Y., & Todorov, A. (2012). Body cues, not facial expressions, discriminate between intense positive and negative emotions. *Science*, 338, 1225–1229.

Bennett, Arnold. (1932). *The journals of Arnold Bennett, 1896–1910.* London: Cassell.

Brehm, J. W. (1999). The intensity of emotion. *Personality and Social Psychology Review*, *3*(1), 2–22. https://doi.org/10.1207/s15327957pspr0301_1

Burgoon, J. K., & Buller, D. B. (1994). Interpersonal deception: Ill-effects of deceit on perceived communication and nonverbal behavior dynamics. *Journal of Nonverbal Behavior*, 18, 155–184.

Chiminello, Anthony. Bridgeworld International. www.bwi.com.au

Clark, I., (2012). Formative assessment: Assessment is for self-regulated learning. *Educational Psychology Review*, *24*(2). doi:10.1007/s10648-011-9191-6

Clay, Rebecca A. (2015). The link between skin and psychology: How psychologists are helping patients with dermatological problems. *American Psychological Association*, *46*(2), 56.

Corstorphine, E. (2006). Cognitive–emotional–behavioural therapy for the eating disorders: Working with beliefs about emotions. *European Eating Disorders Review: The Professional Journal of the Eating Disorders Association*, 14, 448–461.

Craig, A. D. (2002). How do you feel? Interoception: the sense of the physiological condition of the body. *National Review of Neuroscience*, 3, 655–666. doi:10.1038/nrn894

Craig, A. D. (2015). *How do you feel? An interoceptive moment with your neurobiological self.* Princeton, NJ: Princeton University Press. doi:10.1515/9781400852727

Critchley, H. D., & Garfinkel, S. N. (2017). Interoception and emotion. *Current Opinion in Psychology*, 17, 7–14, doi:10.1016/j.copsyc.2017.04.020

Csikszentmihalyi, M. (2008). *Flow: The psychology of optimal experience.* New York: Harper Perennial.

Davies, M., Stankov, L., & Roberts, R. D. (1998). Emotional intelligence: In search of an elusive construct. *Journal of Personality and Social Psychology*, 75, 989–1015.

De Gelder, B., van den Stock, J., Meeren, H. K. M., Sinke, C. B. A., Kret, M. E., & Tamietto, M. (2010). Standing up for the body: Recent progress in uncovering the networks involved in the perception of bodies and bodily expressions. *Neuroscience and Biobehavioral Reviews*, 34, 513–527.

Deikman, A. J. (1982). *The observing self: Mysticism and psychotherapy.* Boston: Beacon Press.

DeSteno, D., Gross, J. J., & Kubzansky, L. (2013). Affective science and health: The importance of emotion and emotion regulation. *Health Psychology*, 32, 474–486.

Diefendorff, J. M., Hall, R. J., Lord, R. G., & Strean, M. L. (2000). Action-state orientation: Construct validity of a revised measure and its relationship to work-related variables. *Journal of Applied Psychology*, 85, 250–263.

Dimitroff, S., Kardan, O., Necka, E., Decety, J., Berman, M., & Norman, G. (2017). Physiological dynamics of stress contagion. *Scientific Reports*, 7, 6168. doi: 10.1038/s41598-017-05811-1

Domes, G., Schulze, L., & Herpertz, S. C. (2009). Emotion recognition in borderline personality disorder: A review of the literature. *Journal of Personality Disorders*, 23, 6–19.

Duncan, B. L., Miller, S. D., Wampold, B. E., & Hubble, M. A. (Eds.). (2010). *The heart & soul of change: Delivering what works in psychotherapy* (2nd ed.). Washington, DC: American Psychological Association.

Dunne, Claire (2015). *Carl Jung, wounded healer of the soul: An illustrated biography.* London: Watkins Media.

Ehlers, A., & Clark, D. M. (2000). A cognitive model of posttraumatic stress disorder. *Behaviour Research and Therapy*, 38, 319–345.

Elfenbein, H. A., & Ambady, N. (2002). On the universality and cultural specificity of emotion recognition: A meta-analysis. *Psychological Bulletin*, 128, 203–235.

Elliot, R., Watson, J. C., Goldman, R. N., & Greenberg, L. S. (2004). *Learning emotion-focused therapy: The process-experiential approach to change.* Washington, DC: American Psychological Association.

Fetterman, A. K., Robinson, M. D., Ode, S., & Gordon, K. H. (2010). Neuroticism as a risk factor for behavioral dysregulation: A mindfulness-mediation perspective. *Journal of Social and Clinical Psychology*, 29, 301–321.

Fieldman Barrett, Lisa, (2017). *How emotions are made: The secret life of the brain.* London: Pan.

Frankl, Viktor E. (2006). *Man's search for meaning* (1946). Boston: Beacon Press.

Fredrickson, B. L. (1998). What good are positive emotions? *Review of General Psychology*, 2, 300–319.

Fredrickson, B. L., & Branigan, C. (2005). Positive emotions broaden the scope of attention and thought-action repertoires. *Cognition & Emotion*, 19, 313–332.

Fredrickson, B. L., Cohn, M. A., Coffey, K. A., Pek, J., & Finkel, S. M. (2008). Open hearts build lives: Positive emotions, induced through loving-kindness meditation, build consequential personal resources. *Journal of Personality and Social Psychology*, 95, 1045–1062.

Fredrickson, B. L., & Kurtz, L. E. (2011). Cultivating positive emotions to enhance human flourishing. In S. I. Donaldson, M. Csikszentmihalyi, & J. Nakamura (Eds.), *Applied positive psychology: Improving everyday life, health, schools, work, and society* (pp. 35–47). Routledge/Taylor & Francis Group.

Fredrickson, B. L., & Levenson, R. W. (1998). Positive emotions speed recovery from the cardiovascular sequelae of negative emotions. *Cognition and Emotion*, 12, 191–220.

Fredrickson, B. L., Mancuso, R. A., Branigan, C., & Tugade, M. M. (2000). The undoing effect of positive emotions. *Motivation and Emotion*, 24(4), 237–258.

Fredrickson, B. L., Tugade, M. M., Waugh, C. E., & Larkin, G. R. (2003). What good are positive emotions in crisis? A prospective study of resilience and emotions following the terrorist attacks on the United States on September 11th, 2001. *Journal of Personality and Social Psychology*, 84, 365–376.

Frijda, N. H. (1986). *The emotions.* Cambridge University Press.

Frijda, N. H., (2007). *The laws of emotion.* Mahwah, NJ: Erlbaum.

Gable, Shelly L., Reis, Harry T., & Elliot, Andrew J. (2000). Behavioral activation and inhibition in everyday life. *Journal of Personality and Social Psychology*, 78(6), 1135.

Gabrielsson, A., & Juslin, P. N. (2003). Emotional expression in music. In R. J. Davidson, K. R. Scherer, & H. H. Goldsmith (Eds.), *Series in affective science. Handbook of affective sciences* (pp. 503–534). New York: Oxford University Press.

Gandhiplein, B. V. Positive Psychology Program. PositivePsychology.org.

Geller, Shari, M., & Greenberg, Leslie, S. (2011). *Therapeutic presence: A mindful approach to effective therapy.* Washington, DC: American Psychological Association.

Geller, Shari (2024). Masterclass: Therapeutic presence and self-compassion for effective therapeutic relationships. www.sharigeller.ca.

Glenberg, A. (2011). Monkey see, monkey do?: The role of mirror neurons in human behavior. *Association for Psychological Science.* www.psychologicalscience.org/news/ releases/monkey-see-monkey-do-the-role-of-mirror neurons-in-human-behavior

Goddard, N. (2015). *Neville Goddard: The complete reader, volume I.* Gearhart, Oregon: Watchmaker Publishing.

Greenberg, L. S. (2017). *Emotion-focused therapy.* Revised edition. American Psychological Association. http://dx.doi.org/10.1037/15971-001.

Greenberg, L. S., (2024). *Shame and anger in psychotherapy.* American Psychological Association. doi.org/10.1037/0000393-001

Greenberg, L. S., Elliott, R. K., & Pos, A. (2007). Emotion-focused therapy: An overview, *European Psychotherapy, 7,* 19–39.

Gross, J. J. (2002). Emotion regulation: Affective, cognitive, and social consequences. *Psychophysiology, 39,* 281–291.

Gross, J. J. (Ed.). (2007). *Handbook of emotion regulation.* New York: Guilford Press.

Gross, J. J., & Muñoz, R. F. (1995). Emotion regulation and mental health. *Clinical Psychology: Science and Practice, 2,* 151–164.

Gross, J. J., & Thompson, R. A. (2007). Emotion regulation: Conceptual foundations. In J. J. Gross (Ed.), *Handbook of emotion regulation* (pp. 3–24). New York: Guilford Press.

Halberstadt, J. B., & Niedenthal, P. M. (2001). Effects of emotion concepts on perceptual memory for emotional expressions. *Journal of Personality and Social Psychology, 81*(4), 587–598. https://doi.org/10.1037/0022-3514.81.4.587

Harte, M. (2019). *Processing emotional pain using emotion focused therapy: A guide to safely working with and resolving emotional injuries and trauma.* Queensland: Australian Academic Press.

Harter, J. K., Schmidt, F. L., & Keyes, C. L. M. (2003). Well-being in the workplace and its relationship to business outcomes: A review of the Gallup studies. In C. L. M. Keyes & J. Haidt (Eds.), *Flourishing: Positive psychology and the life well-lived* (pp. 205–224). *American Psychological Association*. doi.org/10.1037/10594-009

Hatfield, E., Cacioppo, J., & Rapson, R. L. (1994). *Emotional contagion*. New York: Cambridge University Press.

Hayes, S. C., Strosahl, K. D., Wilson, K. G., Bissett, R. T., Pistorello, J., Toarmino, D. (2004). Measuring experiential avoidance: A preliminary test of a working model. *The Psychological Record*, 54, 553–578.

Henssler, J., Andreas Heinz, A., Brandt, L., & Tom Bschor, T. (2019). Review article: Antidepressant withdrawal and rebound phenomena. *Dtsch Arztebl Int.*, *116*(20), 355–361. doi: 10.3238/arztebl.2019.0355

Holtz, Mihaela Ivan. (2025). Creative Minds Psychotherapy. www. creativemindpsychotherapy.com.

Humphreys, K., Minshew, N., Leonard, G. L., & Behrmann, M. (2007). A fine-grained analysis of facial expression processing in high-functioning adults with autism. *Neuropsychologia*, 45, 685–695.

Isaacowitz, D. M., Löckenhoff, C. E., Lane, R. D., Wright, R., Sechrest, L., Riedel, R., & Costa, P. T. (2007). Age differences in recognition of emotion in lexical stimuli and facial expressions. *Psychology and Aging*, 22, 147–159.

Isen, A. M., Daubman, K. A., & Nowicki, G. P. (1987). Positive affect facilitates creative problem solving. *Journal of Personality and Social Psychology*, 52, 1122–1131.

Izard, C. E. (1990). Facial expressions and the regulation of emotions. *Journal of Personality and Social Psychology*, *58*(3), 487–498. https://doi.org/10.1037/0022-3514.58.3.487

Izard, C. E. (1977). *Human emotions*. New York: Plenum Press.

Izard, C. E., Fine, S., Schultz, D., Mostow, A., Ackerman, B., & Youngstrom, E. (2001). Emotion knowledge as a predictor of social behavior and academic competence in children at risk. *Psychological Science*, 12, 18–23.

Jorgensen, P. F. (1998). Affect, persuasion, and communication processes. In P. A. Andersen & L. K. Guerrero (Eds.), *Handbook of communication and emotion: Research, theory, applications, and contexts* (pp. 403–422). San Diego: Academic Press.

Joshi, A.M., Mehta, S.A., Nikhil Pande, N., Mehta, A.O., Kamaljeet Sanjay Randhe, K. S. (2021). Effect of mindfulness-based art therapy (mbat) on psychological distress and spiritual wellbeing in breast cancer patients undergoing chemotherapy. *Indian Journal of Palliative Care*, *27*(4), 552–560. doi: 10.25259/IJPC_133_21

Jung, C. J. (1981). *The archetypes and the collective unconscious*. (1931–1955) New Jersey: Princeton University Press.

Jung, C. J. (1989). *Memories, dreams, reflections* (1962). Recorded and edited by Aniela Jaffe. New York: Vintage.

Jung, C. J. (2009). *The red book: Liber novus* (1915–1932). Trans Mark Kyburz, John Peck and Sonu Shamdasan. Philemon Foundation & W. W. Norton.

Juslin, P. N., & Laukka, P. (2003). Communication of emotions in vocal expression and music performance: Different channels, same code? *Psychological Bulletin*, 129, 770– 814.

Kabat-Zinn, J. (1990). *Full catastrophe living: Using the wisdom of your body and mind to face stress, pain, and illness*. New York: Delacorte.

Kahn, B. E., & Isen, A. M. (1993). The influence of positive affect on variety seeking among safe, enjoyable products. *Journal of Consumer Research*, 20, 257–270.

Kaminski, Patricia. Nurturing the heart-womb: The generative gift of downy avens. fesflowers.com.

Kaminski, P., & Katz, R. Flower essnce repertory. fesflowers.com.

Keltner, D. (1995). Signs of appeasement: Evidence for the distinct displays of embarrassment, amusement, and shame. *Journal of Personality and Social Psychology, 68*(3), 441–454. https://doi.org/10.1037/0022-3514.68.3.441

Kenneth, M., Cramer, K. M., Melanie, D., Gallant, M. D., Michelle, W., Langlois, M. W. (2005). Self-silencing and depression in women and men: Comparative structural equation models. *Personality and Individual Differences, 39*(3), 581–592. https://doi.org/10.1016/j.paid.2005.02.012

Keyes, C. L. M., Wissing, M., Potgieter, J. P., Temane, M., Kruger, A., van Rooy, S. (2008). Evaluation of the mental health continuum–short form (MHC–SF) in Setswana-speaking South Africans. *Clinical Psychology & Psychotherapy, 15*(3), 181–192. doi.org/10.1002/cpp.572

Kilts, C. D., Egan, G., Gideon, D. A., Ely, T. D., & Hoffman, J. M. (2003). Dissociable neural pathways are involved in the recognition of emotion in static and dynamic facial expressions. *Neuroimage*, 18, 156–168.

Kohler, C. G., Walker, J. B., Martin, E. A., Healey, K. M., & Moberg, P. J. (2010). Facial emotion perception in schizophrenia: A meta-analytic review. *Schizophrenia Bulletin*, 36, 1009–1019.

Konttinen, Hanna. (2020). Emotional eating and obesity in adults: The role of depression, sleep and genes. *Proceedings of the Nutrition Society*, 79, 283–289. doi:10.1017/S0029665120000166

Kristeller, J. L. & Miller, D. B. (2011). Mindfulness-based eating awareness training for treating binge eating disorder: The conceptual foundation. *Eating Disorders, 19*(1), 49–61.

Kristeller, J. L. & Wolever, R. Q. (2014). Mindfulness-based eating awareness training: Treatment of overeating and obesity. In *Mindfulness-based treatment approaches* (pp. 119–139). Academic Press.

Lachman, G. (2007). *Rudolf Steiner: An introduction to his life and work.* Edinburgh: Floris Books.

Lamers, S. M., Westerhof, G. J., Bohlmeijer, E. T., ten Klooster, P. M. & Keyes, C. L. (2011). Evaluating the psychometric properties of the mental health continuum–short form (MHC-SF). *Journal of Clinical Psychology, 67*(1), pp.99–110.

Lane, R. D. (2000). Levels of emotional awareness: Neurological, psychological, and social perspectives. In R. Bar-On & J. D. A. Parker (Eds.), *The handbook of emotional intelligence: Theory, development, assessment, and application at home, school, and in the workplace* (pp. 171–191). San Francisco: Jossey-Bass.

Lane, R. D., Ryan, L., Nadel, L., & Greenberg, L. (2015). Memory reconsolidation, emotional arousal, and the process of change in psychotherapy: New insights from brain science. *Behavioural and Brain Sciences*, 38, 1–64.

Lang, P. & Bradley, M. (2010). Emotion and the motivational brain. *Biological Psychology, 84*(3), 437–450. *doi 10.1016/j.biopsycho.2009.10.007*

Linehan, M. M. (1993). *Cognitive-behavioral treatment of borderline personality disorder.* Guilford Press.

McKenzie, S., & Hassed, C. (2012). *Mindfulness for life.* Auckland: Exile.

McKay, M., Rogers, P. D., & McKay, J. (2003). *When anger hurts: Quieting the storm within* (2nd ed.). Oakland, CA: New Harbinger.

Meares, A. (1986). *Cancer: Another way?* Melbourne: Hill of Content.

Meeren, H. K., van Heijnsbergen, C. C., & de Gelder, B. (2005). Rapid perceptual integration of facial expression and emotional body language. *Proceedings of the National Academy of Science USA, 102*(45), 16518–16523. doi: 10.1073/pnas.0507650102.

Meevissen, Y. M., Peters, M. L., & Alberts, H. J. (2011). Become more optimistic by imagining a best possible self: Effects of a two-week intervention. *Journal of Behavior Therapy and Experimental Psychiatry, 42*(3), 371–378.

Mehta, R., Sharma, K., Potters, L., Wernicke, A. G., & Parashar, B. (2019). Evidence for the role of mindfulness in cancer: Benefits and techniques. *Cureus, 11*(5) doi: 10.7759/cureus.4629

Merton, R. K., & Barber, E. (2004). The travels and adventures of serendipity: A study in sociological semantics and the sociology of science. Princeton: Princeton University Press.

Morse, Gardiner. (2006). Decisions and desire. *Harvard Business Review*, https://hbr.org/2006/01/decisions-and-desire

Murray, S. L. (2005). Regulating the risks of closeness: A relationship-specific sense of felt security. *Current Directions in Psychological Science*, 14, 74–78.

Nowicki, S. & Duke, M. P. (1994). Individual differences in the nonverbal communication of affect: The diagnostic analysis of nonverbal accuracy scale. *Journal of Nonverbal Behaviors*, 18, 9–35. https://doi.org/10.1007/BF02169077

Palumbo, Dennis. (2025). https//thecreativemind.net

Parrott, W. G. (1993). Beyond hedonism: Motives for inhibiting good moods and for maintaining bad moods. In D. M. Wegner & J. W. Pennebaker (Eds.), *Handbook of mental control* (pp. 278–305). Prentice-Hall.

Pennebaker, J. W. (1990). *Opening up: The healing power of confiding in others*. New York: William Morrow.

Pennebaker, J. W., & Beall, S. K. (1986). Confronting a traumatic event: Toward an understanding of inhibition and disease. *Journal of Abnormal Psychology*, 95, 27.

Perlman, D. M., Salomons, T. V., Davidson, R. J., & Lutz, A. (2010). Differential effects on pain intensity and unpleasantness of two meditation practices. *Emotion*, *10*(1), 65.

Planck, Max. (1932). *Where is science going?* Trans. James Murphy. New York: Norton & Co.

Raghunathan, R., & Trope, Y. (2002). Walking the tightrope between feeling good and being accurate: Mood as a resource in processing persuasive messages. *Journal of Personality and Social Psychology*, 83, 510–525.

Reinhart, M. (2009). *Chiron and the healing journey: An astrological and psychological perspective*. London: Starwalker Press.

Robbins, Tony. (2024). Where focus goes, energy flows. https://www.tonyrobbins.com/blog/where-focus-goes-energy-flows.

Rockel, A. (2019). *Rogue intensities*. Perth: University of Western Australia Publishing.

Rogers, C. R. (1980). *A way of being: The founder of the human potential movement looks back on a distinguished career*. New York: Houghton Mifflin.

Rowe, G., Hirsh, J. B., & Anderson, A. K. (2007). Positive affect increases the breadth of attentional selection. *Proceedings of the National Academy of Sciences*, 104, 383–388.

Russell, J. A. (1991). Culture and the categorization of emotions. *Psychological Bulletin*, 110, 426–450.

Ryan, R. M., & Deci, E. L. (2001). On happiness and human potentials: A review of research on hedonic and eudaimonic well-being. *Annual Review of Psychology*, 52, 141–166. doi: 10.1146/annurev.psych.52.1.141.

Sabini, J., & Silver, M. (2005). Why emotion names and experiences don't neatly pair. *Psychological Inquiry*, 16, 1–10.

Safran, J. D., & Segal, Z. V. (1990). *Interpersonal process in cognitive therapy.* New York: Basic Books.

Salovey, P., Rothman, A. J., Detweiler, J. B., & Steward, W. T. (2000). Emotional states and physical health. *American Psychologist*, 55, 110–121.

Sapolsky, R. M. (2007). Stress, stress-related disease, and emotional regulation. In J. J. Gross (Ed.), *Handbook of emotion regulation* (pp. 606–615). New York: Guilford Press.

Segerstrom, S. C., Stanton, A. L., Alden, L. E., & Shortridge, B. E. (2003). Multidimensional structure for repetitive thought: What's on your mind, and how, and how much? *Journal of Personality and Social Psychology*, 85, 909–921.

Seligman, Martin E. P. (2002). *Authentic happiness: Using the new positive psychology to realize your potential for lasting fulfillment.* NY: Free Press.

Shapiro, S. L., & Carlson, L. E. (2009). *The art and science of mindfulness: Integrating mindfulness into psychology and the helping professions.* Washington: American Psychological Association.

Shiv, Baba. (2024). More than a feeling: The keys to making the right choice. California: Stanford Graduate School of Business.

Sonnemans J., & Frijda, N. (1994). The structure of subjective emotional intensity. *Cognition and Emotion*, 8, 329–350.

Surawy, C., Hackmann, A., Hawton, K., & Sharpe, M. (1995). Chronic fatigue syndrome: A cognitive approach. *Behaviour Research and Therapy*, 33, 535–544.

Surguladze S. A., Young, A. W., Senior, C., Brébion, G., Travis, M. J. & Phillips, M. L. (2004). Recognition accuracy and response bias to happy and sad facial expressions in patients with major depression. *Neuropsychology*, *18*(2), 212–218. doi: 10.1037/0894-4105.18.2.212.

Tamir, M. (2009). What do people want to feel and why?: Pleasure and utility in emotion regulation. *Current Directions in Psychological Science*, *18*(2), 101–105. https://doi.org/10.1111/j.1467-8721.2009.01617.x

Teasdale, J. D., & Barnard, P. J. (1993). *Affect, cognition, and change: Re-modelling depressive thought.* Lawrence Erlbaum Associates.

Tedeschi, R. G., & Calhoun, L.G. (2009). Posttraumatic growth: Conceptual foundations and empirical evidence. *An International Journal for the Advancement of Psychological Theory*, 15, 1–18. doi. org/10.1207/s15327965pli1501_01

Tolle, Eckart (2018). *The power of now.* Hachette.

Tracy, J. L., & Matsumoto, D. (2008). The spontaneous expression of pride and shame: Evidence for biologically innate nonverbal displays. *Proceedings of the National Academy of Sciences*, 105, 11655–11660.

Tracy, J. L., & Robins, R. W. (2004). Show your pride: Evidence for a discrete emotion expression. *Psychological Science*, *15*(3), 194–197. https://doi.org/10.1111/j.0956-7976.2004.01503008.x

Tracy, J. L., Robins, R. W. & Schriber, R. A. (2009). Development of a FACS-verified set of basic and self-conscious emotion expressions. *Emotion*, *9*(4), 554.

Tsavdari, Evangelina. (2023). Lucis Trust lecture. lucistrust.org.

Van der Kolk, B. (2015) *The body keeps the score: Brain, mind, and body in the healing of trauma.* New York: Penguin Books.

Vine, V., & Aldao, A. (2014). Impaired emotional clarity and psychopathology: A transdiagnostic deficit with symptom-specific pathways through emotion regulation. *Journal of Social and Clinical Psychology*, *33*(4), 319 DOI:10.1521/jscp.2014.33.4.319

Waugh, C. E., & Fredrickson, B. L. (2006). Nice to know you: Positive emotions, self–other overlap, and complex understanding in the formation of a new relationship. *Journal of Positive Psychology*, 1, 93–106.

Wells, M. (2023). *The essential flower essence book: Flower essences for living, healing, personal growth and blossoming.* Melbourne: HSP Health.

Wells, M. (2021). *Embracing the gift of high sensitivity: A guide to living joyfully.* Melbourne: Brolga Publishing.

Westerhof, G. J., & Keyes, C. L. (2010). Mental illness and mental health: The two continua model across the lifespan. *Journal of Adult Development*, *17*(2), 110–119. doi: 10.1007/s10804-009-9082-y.

Wilber, K. (2001). *No boundary: Eastern and Western approaches to personal growth* (2001). Colorado: Shambhala Publications

Willis, J., & Todorov, A. (2006). First impressions: Making up your mind after a 100-ms exposure to a face. *Psychological Science*, 17, 592–598.

Witkower, Z., & Tracy, J. L. (2018). Bodily communication of emotion: Evidence for extrafacial behavioral expressions and available coding systems. *Emotion Review*, 11, 184–193. doi: org/10.1177/1754073917749880

Zeidner, M., Matthews, G., & Roberts, R. D. (2009). What we know about emotional intelligence: How it affects learning, work, relationships, and our mental health. *Boston Review.* doi. org/10.7551/mitpress/7404.001.0001

Zettel, R. D. (2007). *ACT for depression.* Oakland, CA: New Harbinger Publications.

Ziv, A. (1976). Facilitating effects of humor on creativity. *Journal of Educational Psychology*, 68, 318–322.